PSYCHOLOGY OF THE BEATITUDES
by Arpita

Published by
Himalayan International Institute
of Yoga Science and Philosophy
Honesdale, Pennsylvania

ISBN 0-89389-061-8

Library of Congress Catalog Card Number: 79-91136

Copyright 1979
The Himalayan International Institute
of Yoga Science and Philosophy
Honesdale, Pennsylvania 18431

Printed in the United States of America

Foreword

The Sermon on the Mount is one of the most inspiring of all spiritual discourses, and the Beatitudes represent the essence of its teachings. Here, Jesus was speaking to those who were closest and most beloved, to those who could understand his message most clearly—his chosen disciples—and here he expressed the eternal and universal truths which lie behind all religions.

In the Beatitudes Jesus explains what behavior and attitudes are required of those who genuinely wish to enter the path of spirituality. His message transcends any particular religion or culture. It is the very message we are in need of today if we are to transcend our narrow preoccupations and become infused with spiritual understanding.

Though the words Jesus spoke seem to be simple, when we stop to contemplate them we are puzzled, for behind each phrase is a stream of symbolic meaning and implication which may be understood on many levels—and left on our own, we are not able to unfold the implications of Jesus' teachings for our daily lives.

This book, though written simply and clearly, awakens us to many subtleties and profundities in Jesus' words. The author helps us to see how his teaching can transform our daily experiences so that we share in the compassion, peace and understanding which Jesus expressed not only in his words but in his very being.

The author also helps us to become aware of the essential unity between Jesus' ministry and the ancient path of yoga, and by juxtaposing the teachings of these spiritual paths we find that the light shining from each tradition gives clarity to the other. Then, when we penetrate deeper we find that what seemed to be two lights are actually one and the same.

SWAMI AJAYA

Contents

The first version of this book originally appeared as "The Eternal Psychology of the Bible," a series of articles in the *Himalayan News*. *The Jerusalem Bible*, Reader's Edition (New York: Doubleday, 1968) has been used as the reference source throughout except for the Sermon on the Mount in which the King James version has been used.

Introduction

These essays represent some of the learnings I have gleaned from my own experiences and readings as well as from dialogues with myself and with the many who have been catalysts and teachers for me. They are intended to be no more than some impressions I have found helpful in my own struggles toward growth as well as in my intellectual attempts to bring together the yoga and Christian points of view. They are not scholarly or definitive interpretations of the scriptures; I offer them only in the hope that they may serve to support others who are in situations of conflict similar to the ones that I have experienced. I am not a theologian, and I apologize to those more learned than myself who might find fault with the liberties I may sometimes appear to take with Jesus' words.

As I reread the gospels I realized that one of the great difficulties Jesus must have faced in attempting to transmit the nature and attainment of the transcendent reality through words is the fact that they can only suggest the concepts involved. Words are representatives of the rational, linear mode of thinking rather than the intuitive, spatial domain which is the abode of superconscious experiencing. Thus, it seems likely that Jesus used his words as a poet might, and that the essence of their meaning is found not through literal interpretation, but rather through "understanding with the heart."

It is in trying to gaze directly at the star that it fades, in trying to touch the bubble that it bursts, in trying to get close to the bird that it flies away. So then, instead of trying to dissect each letter, or syllable, of Jesus' teachings, appreciating the patterns of the spaces between them and feeling for the message on a higher level will yield more fruitful results. This is because the words of all great religious leaders generate from a source beyond the map of language.

"You are an obstacle in my path because the way you think is not God's way but man's" (Matt. 16:23), said Jesus. Thinking in "man's way," we limit ourselves to our everyday, mundane, temporal consciousness; perceiving reality in broader, deeper terms remains impossible. But by suspending reliance on the familiar, rational framework in which we generally travel, we can choose to rely on our ability to "float" into uncharted waters and experience reality afresh from new perspectives. In other words, the gestalt of an idea may yield a representation which does not resemble its physical counterpart mote for mote, for the whole equals more than the sum of its parts.

It is important to remember this when we deal with Jesus' words. Simple and straightforward, they struck the hearts of those who could receive them, but since he was a mystic, only those who had a notion of Jesus' other-worldly orientation could appreciate his message in all its fullness. Matthew tells us, "He spoke the word to them so far as they were capable of understanding it and . . . explained everything to his disciples when they were alone" (Mark 4:33-34). The crowd was unable to take in all he had to say because it was unable to understand his language fully.

Jesus may have designed his discourses so that this might, in fact, be the case, for his view of life and human nature—that is, his philosophy and psychology—presented a radical shift in the cultural paradigm commonly accepted in his time. His message was one of self-transformation through the power of love and truth, and this was a revolutionary view. In fact, the type of self-improvement program, or therapy, his teachings entailed was totally unacceptable to the elders of his profession.

Jesus' own words and actions, however, which were generated from a highly evolved spiritual state, actually transformed the personalities of others to previously unattained levels of peace and happiness. If followed systematically, they can do that today, for his teachings encourage others to attain these states by being self-reliant, and by giving, and by moving beyond the mundane confines of those societal structures and norms which hamper their personal spiritual growth.

So I have come to consider Jesus to be a fully enlightened spiritual teacher whose words constitute a very sound and practical psychology appropriate for all who seek greater happiness, whether they believe Jesus to be God, an ancient psychotherapist, or a myth.

I appreciate the process of exploration and clarification completing this book has entailed, and I am grateful to my late husband, Tim Thorpe, my parents, Dave and Eloise Harrigan, the residents of the Himalayan Institute, Anne Craig, Dr. S. N. Agnihotri and my other teachers, counselors and friends for their loving support and beneficial interaction, from which I have learned so much. I am especially grateful to my spiritual guide, Sri Swami Rama, who is an endless source of love and inspiration.

I humbly place this little offering at his feet.

ARPITA

I

Be ye therefore perfect . . . .

At an auspicious point in his life Jesus took his closest disciples aside and imparted to them, in a very practical and personal way, the seeds of his teachings. Then carefully relating what they remembered of these instructions, the evangelists recorded them, and they have come down to us as the Sermon on the Mount. These words codify the Christian doctrine, and they are the nectar of Jesus' psychology, embodying the very essence of his philosophy of life. What has come to be known as the Beatitudes are the first part of the Sermon on the Mount, and to be understood properly they must be seen within this context.

The central theme of the Sermon is, "Be ye therefore perfect, even as your Father which is in heaven is perfect" (Matt. 5:48). Consciously or unconsciously, the desire for this perfection smolders in the inner chamber of every human heart. But what does perfection really mean, and how is it attained? Regardless of the culture, or era, into which they were born, those who have deeply investigated human nature and the meaning of life have repeatedly grappled with this question, for it explores the very frontier of human potential. Highly evolved beings, such as Jesus and the mystic sages of the East, represent the "growing tip" of humanity, and having ventured far beyond normal limits, they know the terrain of their own inner domains. Their words therefore provide a map to aid those who wish to travel a similar route.

By comparing the teachings of Jesus to those of the ancient Himalayan sages we obtain a rich view of the transcendental realm in which such mystics dwell and to which those who seek peace and fulfillment may aspire. And the fact that the sayings of these highly evolved beings are so similar establishes the validity of their experiences, for they were attained independently of one another. So let us look at the territory which Jesus and the sages charted as we investigate some of the precepts of their psychologies, beginning with, "Be ye therefore perfect" (Matt. 5:48).

In the Yoga Sutras, the major text of yoga psychology which was codified by Patanjali several centuries before Jesus' birth, it is stated that perfection is attained when the mind becomes as pure as the *atman* (divine soul) itself. The ancient philosopher, Kapila, tells us that perfection is the complete cessation of misery, and writings of yoga psychology explain that perfection is *sat* (immortal life), *chit* (infinite knowledge) and *ananda* (eternal love and bliss). Stated in biblical language, perfection is the Father in heaven—God. *Sat, chit* and *ananda* describe the attributes of God, and the true purpose of life, according to both philosophies, is to find God.

Yoga psychology states that the perfection of the universe is found within every individual and that this indwelling perfection is called *atman*, or the Self. The same concept is also expressed in the Bible when it says, "The Temple of God is sacred, and you are that Temple " (1 Cor. 3:17). Genesis tells us that we are made in the image and likeness of God, and Paul says that we are God's children. If God is omnipresent, then, how can each of us not be permeated with that perfection?

Yoga psychology teaches that because of our ignorance we lose awareness of the reality within and mistakenly identify with the imperfect things of the temporal, material world. Our limited vision sees only the grossest manifestation of that perfection. According to Patanjali, there are five sheaths which surround the reality within: the body, the breath (or energy), the conscious mind, the unconscious mind and transpersonal awareness. These layers hide the divine light shining in everyone as the Self, or soul.

The radiance of this light is everywhere, but it is seen most easily in those evolved individuals who have purified themselves so that the light within shines through. It is the prophets and the sages who manifest the light, who *are* in fact the light. Jesus said, "I am the light of the world" (John 8:12). To take refuge in such a teacher is to take refuge in God.

Nothing in this manifest world (which the sages called illusion, or *maya*) is perfect, and according to yoga psychology it is our involvement with this unreality that causes our misery. The scriptures say, "You will learn the truth, and the truth shall make you free" (John 8:32), but this truth, to the ancients as well as to some modern psychologists, transcends normal concepts of reality. It does not contradict them; it simply goes beyond them.

Mystics have access to this realm of freedom and call it the kingdom of God, or Christ-consciousness. Yoga psychology describes it as *turiya*, the fourth state which lies beyond the three normal states of waking, dreaming and sleeping; gaining access to this state is called variously, personal transformation, or spiritual rebirth—being "born again" into the realm of the Father which can in turn be thought of as either heaven, the beatific vision, self-realization or *samadhi*. In this state one transcends time, space and causation. Multiplicity is obliterated, and those who reside on this level of consciousness experience the true reality in all of its perfection.

According to yoga psychology our current actions are but prefigurings of that perfection which is our true heritage, and in this sense our love for others can be seen as a rehearsal for our love of God. Through human love, we learn love for the divine, for what we are actually loving is the perfection within others. Our attractions are merely unfulfilling substitutes for union with perfection. They are imperfect manifestations of a desire for God disguised as a desire for something else, and our pain and frustration come from attempting to attain perfection from the imperfect. This is like trying to squeeze blood from a turnip. We want others to love us totally and forever, but of course this is not possible; people die, relationships disintegrate.

The Yoga Sutras identify the underlying cause of suffering as ignorance—mistaking the unreal for the real, the temporal for the permanent, the imperfect for the perfect. Besides ignorance, the causes of suffering (called *kleshas*) are attachment, aversion, egoism and the fear of death. It is the purpose of life to understand this clearly and to perfect ourselves, using our time and relationships as opportunities to practice overcoming these *kleshas*—until practice makes perfect.

Besides the *kleshas*, the ancient texts cite laziness and lack of enthusiasm as major obstacles to attaining the goal of perfection. Jesus said, "Hear my words, and act on them" (Luke 6:47), for reality lies beyond doctrine, creeds and philosophy. So when seeking the truth, how can we be satisfied with mere dogma? It is action, experience and inner seeking which are essential to finding reality.

The ancient sages saw attainment of this state of perfection as possible in our present lives, not merely as a reward to be given after death. Jesus said, "I tell you truly, there are some standing here who will not taste death before they see the Son of Man coming with his kingdom" (Matt. 16:28).

Enlightened teachers from numerous spiritual traditions mention many methods for attaining union with the inner perfection which is called God, and all paths lead to this same one source. Even within yoga there are many paths, each suited to various individual temperaments. Karma yoga, for example, prescribes service to humanity; it is overtly represented in the Christian tradition by the many religious orders dedicated to helping the poor, sick and ignorant. Jnana yoga emphasizes discriminating between the real and the unreal—and then renouncing the unreal. This, the intellectual path, is that of such great Christian thinkers as Thomas Aquinas, and the meditative practices it entails are readily apparent in the contemplative orders of Christianity.

Bhakti, the path of devotion, directs the seeker to channel all emotions and desires one-pointedly into love for the Lord and yearning for union with him in keeping with Jesus' saying, "You must love the Lord your God with all your Heart, with all your soul, and with all your mind" (Matt. 22:37). The movingly beautiful expressions of Christian love found in the music and art of the medieval and renaissance periods as well as the ecstatic writings of many saints typify this path of devotion.

Raja yoga, which describes a systematic program for attaining Christ-consciousness, combines elements from all three paths, as do many Christian traditions. For instance, according to raja yoga, purifying the mind through self-control and the observance of ethical values lays the foundation for further development. Then, establishing a schedule of practices to regulate, control and purify the body, the breath and the senses prepares one to calmly focus the mind, with full attention, on the perfect reality within. On the other hand, the Bible instructs, "Be still and know that I am God" (Psalm 46:10). Both traditions maintain that turning the mind inward brings awareness through direct experience of the light within. Meditation deepens devotion and leads to absorption and, finally, to union with that perfection. Love, the lover, and the beloved are then one. People thus become perfect even as their heavenly Father is perfect. As Jesus said,

"God is love, and anyone who lives in love lives in God, and God lives in him" (1 John 4:16).

Both yoga and Christian psychology view the body as a temple which houses this indwelling perfection—that light of divinity which brightly emanates from the hearts of saints but which remains shrouded behind the heavy cloak of human worries in most people. The Yoga Sutras and the Christian aphorisms which Jesus presented as the Beatitudes in the Sermon on the Mount are terse instructions which explain how we can turn our gaze from the darkness which blinds and immobilizes us and realize the brightness of our own divine nature.

Our dilemma is not fear of the dark; it is fear of the light. We cling to the dense shadows of limiting habits and beliefs as if we did not have eyes to see the beatific splendor abiding within our own hearts. As in Plato's metaphor of the cave, we take the shadow images for reality rather than the actual objects revealed by the bright flame of light. Used to the dark, such light hurts our eyes. But as Jesus said, "No one lights a lamp to put it under a tub; they put it on the lampstand where it shines for everyone in the house. In the same way your light must shine . . . " (Matt. 5:15-16).

Shrouded in our familiar darkness, however, we do not perceive the perfect light of our true nature, nor do we believe that we actually *are* that indwelling, all-permeating brilliance of perfection. So in the Beatitudes Jesus provides us with bridges to make our transition from imperfection to perfection. The practices and attitudes he prescribes escort us safely from our familiar, yet unhappy, state of imperfection to our new and blissful state of perfection. The Beatitudes thus serve as reminders and guidelines which nudge and direct our return to the homeland we have forgotten, the perfection of the divine kingdom shining purely and brightly within all of us.

II

You must be born again of the Spirit . . . .
(John 3:3)

Jesus was a master at understanding human nature, and his specialty, as shown in the lessons from the Sermon on the Mount, was transforming personality and building strength of character. His teachings, therefore, give much helpful instruction to those who seek to expand their capacities and attain the farthest reaches of human potential. One much-quoted example of this is the dictum with which Jesus began the Sermon, "Repent, for the kingdom of heaven is close at hand" (Matt. 4:17). This often-misunderstood phrase has been a source of confusion, fear and guilt throughout the ages. But Jesus also said, "Learn from me, for I am gentle and humble in heart, and you will find rest for your souls" (Matt. 11:29).

These two apparently conflicting notions can be reconciled when we recall that Jesus further indicated that the kingdom of heaven is within us, and therefore ever-present. In other words, we encompass that perfection always and have only to become aware of it; the capacity to attain self-realization, to identify with what the yogis call the *atman*, is constantly ours. So Jesus' advice to those who would experience this is to "repent." This does not necessarily mean, as so many have interpreted it, that we are evil and ought to feel guilty; it might very well mean simply that we could benefit by reconsidering the consequences of our habitual patterns of behavior and, regretting where they have led us (or failed to lead us), contemplate more efficient avenues to happiness.

The practice of replacing deleterious habits for more beneficial ones is an essential technique in yoga psychology. It results in a different mental outlook, free from the rut we have dug and continue to deepen by continued use. Thus, this word *repent*, which at first may seem like a threat or an indictment, can be appreciated instead as an instructive and loving recommendation. *Repent* in this sense can mean to decide to change and to maintain a persistent effort in the chosen direction.

Jesus' moral teaching is based not on outward rules but on inner principles. He told his disciples, "If your virtue goes no deeper than that of the scribes and Pharisees, you will never get into the kingdom of heaven" (Matt. 5:20). These groups were reknowned for their literal and picayune interpretation of the law, although they were often thought to be exemplary adherents of their faith. But Jesus seems to indicate that their rote behavior is superficial and unproductive. They miss the point.

Jesus always emphasized the emotional tone underlying observable behavior rather than the form itself, and he aimed at strengthening character by means of love, service and a drive to self-knowledge. These are also the tools of bhakti, karma and jnana yoga—devotion, action and contemplation. Patanjali in the Yoga Sutras also stresses the spirit rather than the letter of the law when he describes the ten virtues that will enhance spiritual growth, the *yamas* and *niyamas*. According to these, one must abstain from harming others, from falsehood, from theft, from incontinence and from greed. Keeping the observances of purity, contentment, mortification, study and striving toward God is also helpful. But even so, an action in itself is neither intrinsically good nor bad. The consequences of one's behavior are either beneficial or detrimental to growth. That is all.

Rejection, ridicule, shame and fear do not motivate sincere seekers. Instead, what has been called "a naked intent unto God" spurs them to recondition and reeducate themselves intrinsically in preparation for spiritual development. By learning to have control over their senses and appetites, they strive to tame and pacify the desires which urge them away from this goal, for they want to store the psychic energy that is usually released through preestablished patterns of sense and ego gratification, and rechannel it. Thus, they intensify the force with which they pursue attainment of finer levels of consciousness.

In the Sermon on the Mount Jesus instructs his followers to set their hearts on the heavenly kingdom and not to concern themselves with the body (such sensory withdrawal is called *pratyahara* in yoga psychology). Thus, by focusing on spiritual desire, seekers slowly establish and strengthen new patterns by habitual repetition of more productive behavior as well as through nonperformance of the old ways which they hope to extinguish.

Dealing with the obstacles to growth require constant effort. As Jesus said, "A man's enemies will be those of his own household" (Matt. 10:36). So too in the *Bhagavad Gita*, another important yoga text, the hero, Arjuna, had to engage in a war between members of his own family. Interpreting these metaphors psychologically, it is apparent that the conflict is an internal one, dealing with one's ever-familiar and limiting habits of thought and emotion. Many of these are hard to eliminate because they were meticulously developed in the past as helpful allies, serving to defend us from threatening feelings, realizations and interactions. But even though they eventually outlive their usefulness, and now limit our progress, we still tend to remain attached to them, and thus they become handicaps.

Patanjali tells us that to be free from thoughts that distract us, thoughts of an opposite kind should be cultivated. Jesus tells us, "Come to terms with your opponent in good time" (Matt. 5:25). So as soon as we can recognize an old inner tendency which now opposes our growth, we would do well to observe it, understand its function, devise a more appropriate means of dealing with the issue and replace the old pattern with a new one.

This results in a gradual, gentle evolution in which the major field of change is not so much overt behavior as it is the covert mental/emotional activity which directs it. In this way desires eventually shift, on the subtle level, until actions become congruent with the spiritual aspirations of the seeker. Old habits may sometimes stubbornly surface, but they will merely pass through and dissipate if they are not reinforced, choked down or clung to. This develops the attitude of non-attachment, an essential mental stance in yoga psychology.

Resolving conflicts in this way defuses their power over us, and making the conscious choice to observe and replace restrictive habits finds eloquent support in Jesus' words, "It will do you less harm to lose one part of you than to have your whole body thrown into hell" (Matt. 5:30). Identifying and letting go of one's psychic armor can be a frightening and painful process, however.

But if we manage to do it we will find that in the absence of our old automatic responses we are free to act with greater creativity and responsibility. Thus, we become more spontaneous and have a greater field of choice within which to move. And this freedom gives us increased energy with which we can discover our true selves. Breaking through this shell is the natural process of development.

This does not mean that we must overthrow the past entirely. Jesus said, "I have not come to abolish the Law of the Prophets . . . but to complete them" (Matt. 5:17). We do not have to destroy either the past or the personality in order to reach greater emotional maturity; we can use what has gone before as the foundation on which further growth can be formed. It is counterproductive to try to either destroy or deny the past, or to ruminate on it, or to cling to it. We can simply accept it, make use of our strengths and go on to create the best present possible. It is not necessary to endlessly analyze what has gone before. The important thing is to identify our future spiritual goals and to be aware of our present capacity. "Leave the dead to bury their dead" (Luke 9:60), said Jesus.

Since personality is a composite of little habits, consistent repetition of beneficial activities (which are mutually exclusive of the detrimental ones) will eventually shape a new way of relating to self and others. Consistent, gentle effort and an attitude of self-acceptance and forgiveness are essential. One cannot push a river; one can merely trust its forward-flowing tendency. "Do what you can, and be grateful for what you can do" is a helpful motto. Accepting our "sins" as obstacles, as the yogis do, rather than crimes can help us continue forward with increased determination instead of being paralyzed by self-recriminating hopelessness.

It is futile to think that a "Thou shalt not" mentality, or legalistic admonitions, will succeed in transforming the personality. This will only lead to repression or a rebellious expression of the desire which one is trying to overcome—and when a desire is repressed, it is still in control. We do not have conscious awareness of its force and cannot prevent it from dictating behavior. The other side of the coin, and just as hazardous, is unrestrained expression of all desires. Instead, we would do best to become aware of our inner urges and accept their presence while regulating their expression. One controls their influence by training them to manifest only in certain ways and at certain times and places.

For those who are pursuing the goal of self-actualization, the best attitude to take is that behavior which is not beneficial to our growth is simply not within the realm of possibility. If it is not on the menu, then it cannot be selected. Why go out and eat ashes when there is fragrant soup right before us?

Yet if we still have an appetite for ashes, we may need to experience their unpleasant effects for ourselves before we are ready to select something more nutritious and pleasing, and then it is sometimes helpful to sanction and schedule gratification of some impulses. This is quite healthy. The degree to which we limit our expression depends on the style of life we have chosen and the goals we have set.

In learning to redirect our emotional impulses, there are a few other techniques that may be helpful. One way is to allow, when necessary, for the expression, or venting, of pent-up emotions (such as crying when we are sorrowful). Another way is to engage in self-analysis and dialogue in order to more clearly assertain our own dynamics and blocks. The third way is to regularly spend time in quiet contemplation, simply allowing our desires to surface and pass through our awareness.The second two are techniques of raja yoga in which the cultivation of non-attachment, self-observation and meditation are basic to the process of growth.

Possibly one of the most effective ways to avoid being tossed by unbridled urges is by sublimating them—that is, by harnessing their energy into positive action for the benefit of others. This involves a kind of transmutation of energy. The force is still there, but it is manifested in a different form. This new behavior, in turn, reinforces and shapes the self-concept that is being developed. In addition, we reap the benefits of increased concentration and vitality.

In pursuing the goal of self-realization, however, it is the fundamental emotional attitude which matters most, for that is what motivates thought and behavior and, thus, bit by bit, brings about a transformation of character. The process of letting go of the maladapative facets while establishing more productive facets of personality is not only fundamental to yoga psychology, it is also the key to Jesus' psychology when he says, "Anyone who loses his life for my sake will find it" (Matt. 16:25). This notion is epitomized in the Sermon on the Mount when he says, "I have come not to abolish but to complete [the Law]" (Matt. 5:17), and, "No one can be the slave of two masters" (Matt. 6:24). We must build on our strengths and be willing to let go of conflictual attachments in order to attain a rebirth into greater spiritual maturity.

III

Blessed are the poor in spirit . . . .

The Beatitudes constitute the core of the Sermon on the Mount. Comprising a beautiful prose poem, they not only praise those who have attained the spiritual heights, they also offer the seeker instruction in how to transform himself. In the sense that they deal with the essence rather than the letter of the law, these lessons are reminiscent of other similar teachings such as the Ten Commandments, Buddha's eightfold path and the ten restraints and observances (*yamas* and *niyamas*) described in the Yoga Sutras. They can be viewed as spiritual seeds to be contemplated and pondered and, once grasped, they can be put into action and applied to daily life. As is true of all great literature, these short sayings can be experienced on three levels: the literal, the metaphorical and the transcendental.

The first Beatitude, "Blessed are the poor in spirit: for theirs is the kingdom of heaven" (Matt. 5:3) summarizes the mental attitude necessary for the transformation of personality. Analyzing these words as poetry, their deeper meaning begins to reveal itself. *Blessed* means having been bestowed with divine favor, or touched by the love of God. It is sometimes translated as *happy*, or *fortunate*. The blessed are holy and pure and reside in a state of endless bliss. Having been given the gift of grace from God, they are able to direct this grace to others. *Poor* means those who have virtually nothing. Lacking the resources to live even minimally comfortable lives, they have no unnecessary possessions, owning only that which is essential for survival. They lead simple, basic lives and can easily discriminate between what they really need and what they can do without. They are motivated by need, not whim. The poor often have no easy way to support themselves and must spend their efforts in long, hard hours of work. Frequently they must depend for their survival on the generosity of others, by begging. *Spirit* is that which is beyond the physical, material plane. It is the life principle, or animating influence, which is beyond the body and mind. *Spirit* can also mean a particular frame of mind, or temperament.

The "poor in spirit," then, are those who, realizing their need, seek only that which is necessary for their spiritual survival. They carry nothing superfluous with them on their journey through life, but keep themselves empty and open so that they may be filled with spiritual nurturants.

They are not satisfied with material, or temporal, good, so they come to God with empty begging bowls.

Jesus said, "God is spirit, and those who worship must worship in spirit and truth" (John 4:24). The poor in spirit rely on God's charity for their spiritual survival, and this gives direction to their lives. Those who have nothing, spiritually, admit their need and have made room for God to dwell within them.

Spiritual poverty, then, is much different from material poverty although they sometimes go hand in hand. Jesus teaches that "it is easier for a camel to pass through the eye of a needle than for a rich man to enter the kingdom of heaven" (Matt. 19:24), and the great yoga philosopher, Shankara, states that there is no way of attaining immortality through wealth; Luke writes, "But alas for you who are rich: you are having your consolation now" (Luke 6:24); and the Vedas teach that neither by rituals, nor by progeny, nor by riches, but by renunciation alone can immortality be attained.

Jesus, too, advocated renunciation of material attachments. In demonstrating how to overcome our limitations, he instructed, "Shoulder my yoke and learn from me" (Matt. 11:29), and, "My yoke is easy and my burden light" (Matt. 11:30). But his requirements sound rather strenuous, for he also declared, "If anyone wants to be a follower of mine, let him renounce himself and take up his cross and follow me" (Matt. 16:25), and, "None of you can be my disciple unless he gives up all his possessions" (Luke 14:33), and "Take nothing for the journey" (Luke 9:3), and, "Enter by the narrow gate" (Matt. 7:13). Taken at face value, these requirements seem impossible for one who lives in the world, but taken in a more universal sense they prescribe the proper frame of mind needed to attain the transcendent levels of consciousness typical of the self-realized, integrated personality. In modern terms these words might be interpreted to say, "Let go of your old self-concepts, your old patterns of behavior and your limited frameworks for perceiving the world. Accept the fact that your destiny and purpose is to become fully actualized, and strive steadfastly toward this end, eliminating all distractions." Jesus pointed out that "the worries of this world and the lure of riches chokes the word" (Matt. 13:22).

Jesus' teachings, as well as yoga psychology thus tell us that wealth is neither good nor bad; it is one's attitude toward material possessions which matters. Deep attachment to the things of the material world is thus seen to burden the spirit and render it incapable of soaring to spiritual heights. The desire for physical objects must therefore be renounced on the spiritual level so that the spirit will not be distracted but will seek only that which it truly needs. This is not to say that we should not use material things or pleasures; it is simply better not to rely on them, become addicted to them or identify with them.

Our attachments may be to objects, pleasures, thoughts, actions, emotions or desires. In our ignorance we identify ourselves with these distractions, and although it may appear that we therefore have a great deal—in reality, we own nothing. Everything is on loan to us in this life. Wealth, position, education, petty concerns—even our bodies—amount to nothing in the long run. They are temporary and insignificant. So the seeker is better off to jettison attachment to everything that can stand in the way of personal growth. When Christ called the humble, unlearned fishermen to follow him they, being poor in spirit, gladly followed, but when he called the rich young man, he "went away sad, for he was a man of great wealth" (Matt. 19:22).

Possessions do not mean just material wealth; they also include the preconceived ideas, the daily dreams, the sensual pleasures, the attachments to institutions, the desire for exciting experiences, the worry over the opinions of others and the sense of self-importance which keeps us chained to the mundane level and clouded in illusion. The hardest things to let go of are frequently our own negative tendencies, identified in yoga psychology as the causes of suffering, the *kleshas*—ignorance, addiction, aversion, egoism and fear.

In addition to referring to a lack of, or an

attachment to things of the world, the term *spiritual poverty* also has another meaning. It is said that the first step to knowledge is to admit our ignorance; likewise, the first step to spiritual wealth is to admit our spiritual poverty. From a spiritual perspective we are all paupers and orphans, and yet we are all heir to the vast wealth of our heavenly father and our divine mother. According to yoga psychology, in clinging to the small change of false identification with the objects of the world, we are distracted from our true purpose and thereby remain ignorant of our birthright and home. However, if we declare our spiritual bankruptcy through admitting that we really have nothing, that we are ignorant and that we cannot survive without spiritual nourishment, then we may be filled with grace and peace.

Admitting our spiritual poverty, however, does not mean indulging in self-condemnation. To objectively assess our condition is to be truthful, and this means honesty, not self-rebuke. When we cry out in need and realize where our salvation lies, then help will be forthcoming. As Jesus said, "Ask, and it will be given to you" (Matt. 7:7).

So we must seek spiritual wealth with the humility of a beggar. In the Yoga Sutras Patanjali instructs us to come to a spiritual teacher with only three things: reverence, a willingness to serve and inquisitiveness regarding spiritual matters. Shankara tells us that after we have put ourselves in a state of perfect renunciation and have found a sage capable of imparting instruction, we should learn from him or her, making the teachings a part of ourselves and identifying with our teacher and with God. Thus, to transform ourselves, we must be willing to shed our old skins because, as Jesus said, "Nobody pours new wine into old wineskins" (Mark 2:22). We should seek spiritual wealth with an attitude of spiritual poverty, being receptive, selfless, pure and unaffected by attachments.

Like the poor, we must one-pointedly and energetically seek that which we need in order to survive. We have no time for distractions such as pride, jealousy, desires for things of little substance and other petty concerns. We should be pure, simple and determined, and we should remain uninfluenced by our mundane surroundings. Jesus said to come to him as little children, with trust, love and openness. He assures us that he will then care for us even as the Father provides for the lilies of the field and the birds of the air. Then, when we attain this level of spiritual poverty, the kingdom of heaven, or enlightenment, will be ours. This is the path of saints who, like Francis of Assisi, literally threw their worldly wealth out of the window.

Viewing the meaning of this Beatitude in its widest sense, a still broader meaning unfolds. Patanjali tells us that the highest state of spiritual development, called *samadhi*, is the cessation of thought waves in the mind. In seedless *samadhi* even the one undistracted thought of God is transcended, and the spirit resides in a state of being one with God. This is the true spiritual poverty in which one is so absolutely devoid of anything that one is at once full of everything: the void is the One; the emptiness is the fullness. Viewed in this light, the first Beatitude does not seem quite so abstruse after all. It means exactly what it says—when one is completely empty, then enlightenment occurs.

This is the goal of meditation, and the Yoga Sutras convey this same message. As Patanjali tells us, that which fills our minds consists of right knowledge, wrong knowledge, verbal delusion, sleep and memory. To be free from the thoughts that distract us from the spiritual realm, thoughts of the spirit within must be cultivated. These are nourished by practicing stillness and non-attachment, and meditation is the basic tool for accomplishing this. Through meditation, one closes off the sensory-motor mind, allows the unconscious to flow out, expands the ego and comes in touch with the guidance of the inner voice.

According to yoga science, then, an attitude of aloofness to things of the world is beneficial, for although we are in the world, we would be better off to remain above the distractions which draw us away from spirituality. This is what is meant by "being in the world, and yet above it." Patanjali also says that mistaking the changing, physical aspects of existence for the real and the permanent is called ignorance, and he adds that to identify consciousness with that which merely reflects consciousness is egoism. He compares a mind which is cleared of all thought waves to a pure crystal which takes on the color of the object nearest to it. Thus, the spirit identifies with the object of its concentration.

We are therefore advised to take caution regarding what we concentrate on and desire. For, as Jesus says, "Where your treasure is, there will your heart be also" (Matt. 6:21). Perfection may be obtained by concentrating only on the perfect, but if we fill our minds on a wealth of material concerns, we may be tempted away from the truth. In other words, it is through the power of the will that we reap the fruits of our desires, be they beneficial or detrimental to our personal growth.

More pointedly, Patanjali tells us, for example , that when people become steadfast in the abstension from theft, all wealth will come to them. This paradox is also expressed in the Bible, "Set your heart on his kingdom first . . . and all these other things shall be given you as well" (Matt. 6:33), and, "For the least among you all, that is the one who is great" (Luke 9:48). In other words, by cultivating poverty, one attains great wealth. As an Indian sage once described it, "I left a few paltry rupees and a few petty pleasures for a cosmic empire of endless bliss . . . . The shortsighted worldly folk are the real renunciates. They relinquish an unparalleled divine possession for a poor handful of earthly toys!"*

The *sadhus*, who keep only a loincloth and a water jug and never stay in the same place for longer than three nights, are weaning themselves from relying on outer things so that their journey within will be easier. The vows of poverty which are taken in most monastic orders are more than a practice in discipline; they also aid the student by eliminating the distractions of the material plane and thereby freeing energy which can be used for spiritual matters. They understand that, "A man's life is not made secure by what he owns" (Luke 12:15). The great mystics know that when the spirit is devoid of all else, the kingdom of heaven abounds. When all else falls away, we realize the presence of the eternal beyond within us. This is how the poor in spirit possess the kingdom of heaven.

* Paramahansa Yogananda. *Autobiography of a Yogi* (Los Angeles: Self Realization Fellowship, 1973), p. 75.

IV

Blessed are they that mourn . . . .

The second Beatitude is, "Blessed are they that mourn: for they shall be comforted" (Matt. 5:4). Mourning is our response to losing something which we hold dear to us, something with which we identify. At different times we mourn for different things, and the more precious the thing we miss is to us, the more intense is our mourning. Sometimes we mourn only for an object or behavior we did not keep; sometimes it is for the house, job or lover we could no longer have or for the pet who has met an ill fate. Sometimes it is for our own youth and dreams which are slowly fading away. Generally, however, when we think of mourning, we are thinking of the suffering which follows the death of someone very close to us.

When we are mourning we are steeped in anguish. We think constantly of that which we have lost, and we long to be reunited. We feel that nothing else can give us comfort. Everything but that seems stale, and we feel alone, without purpose, and confused. The world offers no solace; the roles we once played seem useless; and we find ourselves turning ever more inward.

The thought of a "homecoming" with our loved one fills our hearts and minds—that and a flurry of questions which attempt to make sense of our present state of misery. We are down to the nub, encountering alone the meaning of existence. "Why has this thing happened? Where has my loved one gone? What can be worth doing now?" It is as if a vital part of us has been rudely ripped away—and yet we live on, crippled and disconnected. A gaping wound is our constant focus of awareness.

As though we too had ceased existence in this world, our spirits search the cosmos for our beloved. We yearn for our own release from everyday existence; surely death would relieve our suffering, and we could rest in its sweet embrace with our beloved. How can we go on without that union? What use is it to continue in this emptiness? But here we remain, on the other side of the border, wondering why survivors should be considered fortunate. Mechanically, we continue to perform our duties, to feign life, but our hold on this mundane plane is light.

We are tempted to retreat to our inner world of fantasy, to deny our fate and to live with old memories and dreams. We savor every good moment from the past and regret every wasted one and every selfish act.

We become protective of our private world, afraid that others may intrude, afraid lest they too depart, taking part of us with them, for as the yogis say, it is attachments which makes us lonely. And yet we long for their loving companionship, for that soothing intimacy we once had. We want to withdraw from others, yet we want to be enveloped in their love. We want to be comforted, to weep as Jesus did at Lazarus' death, and to talk ceaselessly of our dead loved one and of our feelings, yet others seem uncomfortable with our grief, and so we remain silent.

Even the happy memories bring sadness. Commonplace scenes and familiar objects trigger our grief as waves of sorrow, waves of anger, suddenly surge within us with overpowering force. Blaming ourselves and others, we find relief from our guilt and rage only in interludes of depression or brief distraction. We grasp for explanations, for some reason that can make the tragedy more acceptable. But even plausible rationales do not reconcile our grief.

Despite what others may try to do to help, there is no escape from our torment. Nobody can take our pain away, for it runs too deep for anyone else to touch. We at last resign ourselves to the reality of our loss, and quietly, slowly, in darkness and solitude, the hard work of mending gradually begins. Fiber by fiber, a new thread must be formed. The fabric must be rewoven, but it will never again be the same.

We want to begin again, to be renewed, but we do not want to let go of that which we once had. We are forced to rely on our own resources regardless of how much we may fight against this reality, for only we can create the solution to our dilemma. But as the months go by time mercifully filters some of the pain, and we who mourn adjust to our loss, each in our own different way.

Some slowly put the main pieces back together and manage to carry on by closing off and blocking sad memories as thoroughly as possible. They wrap themselves in a layer of gauze, and numb to their own true feelings and to contact with life, they accept respite by anesthetizing their awareness of themselves, not even feeling the vague, dazed state in which they exist. Others turn for solace to diversions such as travel, business, spending, drinking and social relationships. They busily create a flurry of intense situations in order to distract their attention from the more pressing dilemma in which they are caught.

For some, the mourning never stops, and they become bitter, falling into a self-pitying grief and remaining constantly depressed, caustic or even vengeful. Rage, turned inward or outward, abides as the focus of their lives. Some others continually relieve their most terrible moment, passively awaiting a magic solution, using their emotions to draw pity and support from others so they themselves can remain dependent and helpless.

A few, on the other hand, experience a kind of awakening and begin life afresh. But having viewed the world from a different perspective, they are not able to return to a life of strictly secular concerns or follow their ordinary patterns of existence. The everyday world seems like a cardboard stage prop compared to that glimpse of eternity they touched as they helplessly watched all that held meaning for them slip into the beyond. They have seen through the veil of *maya* and know that reality is eternal spirit, not transient matter. No mundane pleasures can give them comfort; they must also seek the beyond.

There is nothing else left to do. They realize that their only refuge exists nowhere in this world. They have felt an instant of deeper reality, and the illusion of life's melodrama is over for them, for they know it for the sham it is and must look beyond the setting, the script, the makeup and the props to understand the underlying reality it holds.

Their suffering drives them to learn the truth, and with dedication they strive for union with it. They hold constant awareness of the precious, fragile quality of life and of the permanence and strength of the spirit. Appreciating the time and talents given to them, they find meaning in attempting to accomplish some useful task in this brief space left to them.

Pain has thus made a needle of what was once

a pin, and they are open to be threaded and used for a different purpose. They allow their sorrow to act as a positive force, helping to fill in their loss, healing them, and guiding them to reshape their tangled lives. Like children, they face the world—open, defenseless, and trusting—for surely the greatest pain has already been incurred, and no other can really threaten them. Having gazed through the portals of death, they realize it is only a transition, and they do not fear it.

So accepting their vulnerability to life's hardships, they relinquish all fantasies of having control over the universe, and by thus letting go, they somehow gain strength, courage, nurturance and hope. Their pain has brought them brightness and beauty, for they have been awakened to a richer existence. They turn self-destructiveness into self-reliance, weakness into power. They find their way through suffering by coming in touch with their inner wisdom as well as by coming to terms with their plight and by accepting their duty. With honesty, confrontation, acceptance and engagement, they come through the ordeal by experiencing their feelings fully while maintaining their focus on a deeper reality. And thus they turn tragedy into one of the most dynamic and growth-enhancing periods of their lives.

This world has been called a vale of tears, and in the second Beatitude Jesus speaks with compassion of our plight, assuring us that there will be an end to suffering. His was a gospel of joy, and he sought to spread love wherever he found misery. Healing and teaching, he lived to give comfort and to show the tools we need to overcome grief, for in a very real sense we are all mourners. We all know that something is missing in our lives, and we attempt to fill this gap in the same way mourners do, groping for any speck of comfort we can find.

Despite our sometimes desperate attempts to be happy, however, our lives usually remain devoid of purpose and meaning, and the saddest aspect of this existential dilemma of emptiness is that most of us do not even know what it is that we are mourning. Further, we do not realize that we actually have the capacity to be reunited with it. We have lost our way and forgotten our home, but the definite impression that there is something better than what we now have remains, making us dissatisfied and restless.

According to yoga psychology, our misery is caused by separation from this something better, the Self, and the separation exists because of our rigid ego and our attachment to things of little consequence. The source of these desires is our ignorance of what lies beyond this physical realm. We think reality exists only on this plane, and caught in the illusion of *maya*, we look for happiness in the wrong places, in the wrong ways. We let trinkets distract us from finding our inheritance of vast wealth. The more we separate ourselves from these attachments, however, the freer we are from the suffering associated with them. The more we lose, the more we will be comforted. Although we may feel as though we are really very distant from our spiritual home, all its bliss and comfort actually dwell within us, and the more intensely we long for union with it, the more quickly we will realize it.

In spiritual mourning, we grieve for our most precious loss, and although this parallels the symptoms of mourning for a lost spouse or child, it is even more intense, because union with the object of our love in this case is our destiny and our true nature. Separation from this is separation from ourselves; it is a living death. Viewed from this broader perspective, the mourners that Jesus refers to in the second Beatitude seem to be those who are aware that their suffering is caused by their separation from what Jesus calls the Lord thy God and what Patanjali refers to as the true Self which dwells within and beyond. They know what they are missing, and they strive to regain it.

This special mourning is essential for attaining spiritual happiness, and it is therefore called "blessed." It marks a point in our individual evolution, a "dark night of the soul," when our suffering is unconsoled by anything except the vision of the beyond, of being one with the One. That yearning alone fills our mind, heart and soul, and every action is performed as an attempt to grow closer to our indwelling Beloved.

Our unhappiness, then, is a signal that we are

lacking something essential. It is an alarm loving-
ly rousing us to persistently seek our spiritual
survival. If we are sensitive to it, it will lead us to
the comfort we are seeking. Often, though, we
have to go through much darkness and misery to
find our way. Only after all seems lost, after we
have tried everything and are still unhappy,
after we have given up attachment to each in-
effective method of relieving our anxiety and
loneliness—only then do we recognize the path
and prepare ourselves for the long journey home.

Yoga psychology explicitly teaches that at
death the body's breath and conscious mind
cease to exist, while the Self, the transpersonal
awareness, and the unconscious mind and conscience travel on through a series of incarnations
until final liberation, or *samadhi,* is reached. In
the Christian doctrine such an outlook is not
explicitly stated, but can easily be inferred.
Here, the soul is said to leave the body at death,
and the final goal is heaven, but some of Jesus'
words indicate that the concept of reincarnation
was accepted by his followers who readily dis-
cussed the notion that John the Baptist was
Elija returned. The ideas of limbo, purgatory and
hell could also metaphorically refer to what in
yoga is thought of as the space between lifetimes;
they could also refer to the future lifetimes of
suffering one must experience before attaining
sufficient purity to reach heaven, or *samadhi,*
when the chain of rebirths is broken.

Viewing life from this perspective, death and spiritual striving take on broader meaning. For instance, according to this paradigm we use each lifetime to set up the experiences we need in order to work through our blocks to growth and to pay off whatever moral debts we may have previously incurred. According to yoga, we actually attract and unconsciously create such situations in order to learn the lessons essential to our spiritual development. Sometimes these lessons involve the death of someone very dear to us, and sometimes they focus on very intense yearning for union with our spiritual lord—the One beyond within.

Jesus as well as the ancient yoga masters assure us that fervent spiritual yearning will be rewarded, but to reach that level, we must "die" to this worldly plane through non-attachment, virtuous actions and love for God and others. But since we are all mourners, we can also all be comforters, and this helps us on our journey. All else will only hold us back; it must be left behind. This realization, the process of reconstruction and the sense of purpose are the gifts given to mourners. Accepting this, the joyous dawn of spiritual light will begin to grow within us, and we may bask in the warm glow of its nurturing love. This is the blessed and comforting reunion for which we all mourn and to which we are all heir. As Jesus said, "Your sorrow will turn to joy" (John 16:20), and as the Psalms sing, "Those who went sowing in tears now sing as they reap" (Psalms 126:5).

V

Blessed are the meek. . . .

The third Beatitude Jesus delivered in the Sermon on the Mount was, "Blessed are the meek: for they shall inherit the earth" (Matt. 5:5). This quiet little verse is a virtual symphony of spiritual wisdom, and by tuning into it, we can achieve Christ-consciousness. Its full import, however, frequently escapes the ears of the modern listener, for the cacophony of brash noises to which we are attuned in our hectic lifestyles clashes with the unassuming melody of this delicate line. Meekness is hardly considered to be a virtue in our aggressive, "go-get-'em" culture. In fact, meekness is now thought of as a derogatory term, used synonymously with *passive* and *weak,* and why would anyone actually want to cultivate an attribute which most people would seek the aid of psychotherapists to over-come? To appreciate the beauty of meekness, we must suspend our initial aversion to its connotations and assume that Jesus chose to reiterate this

Old Testament quote because its effect would enhance our personal growth.

Let us accept, then, that the word *meek* has currently fallen upon hard times, that its true meaning has become distorted. Consider also that this term is also translated as *gentle* in some versions of the Bible. Jesus was certainly not encouraging his followers to become spiritless and timid. Rather, by advocating meekness, he was urging us to adopt the most disciplined and powerful attributes of the spiritual seeker: self-surrender, egolessness, non-attachment, humility and faith—virtues highly valued in yoga psychology also. Meekness entails strength, will, courage and control of the emotions. This is no namby-pamby quality—it is an active, determined, dynamic, positive force. It looks passive only to those who limit their view to the external; the activity is within.

First, meekness entails surrendering oneself to the higher will. As Jesus said, "My food is to do the will of the one who sent me, and to complete his work" (John 4:34). This is not a passive giving up, but a faithful letting go—a letting go of the fear, egoism, resistance and doubt which weigh us down. In yoga psychology meekness, or self-surrender, is a strategy for overcoming the *kleshas*, the causes of suffering. It is like water, gently conforming and flowing within the contours given it. Its strength lies in the fact that nothing can check it; nothing can push it; it will always find its own way. Eventually, even the earth itself will give way beneath its determined striving for its destination. Water allows itself to find its own destiny. In yielding to its own nature, its innate tendency is released, and strong, it merges with its goal.

Learning to be meek is like learning to swim. At first it looks impossible, and if we fight the water or stiffen, we will sink. But when we trust ourselves, relax and let the water support us, our own potential is released—and we float. Then, with awareness and conscious effort, we become more adept in moving through the water, and we use its current to guide us. Thus, in yielding to our natural tendency to float, or to be meek, we develop the means to flow toward our own destination of inner perfection. Only our struggling and resistance, caused by the hardening of our ego, constricts us and causes us to sink.

Accepting the discipline of meekness does not break the spirit. Rather, it cracks the ego so the spirit can soar free. Taking on the stance of student, child and servant releases us to see every situation as an opportunity to learn, enjoy and serve. It opens us to the flow of intuition and makes us unconquerable, for where there is no resistance, there is no conflict. The meek are quiet, gentle, simple and loving. They do their work as best they can, as the *Bhagavad Gita* admonishes, and demand nothing, nor do they expect anything in return. It is the skillful performing of the task which holds its own intrinsic reward and benefits others. Jesus said, "If anyone wants to be first, he must make himself last of all and servant to all" (Mark 9:35), and "For everyone who exalts himself will be humbled, and the man who humbles himself will be exalted" (Luke 14: 11), and, "The last will be first, and the first, last" (Matt. 20:16). The meek say, "We are merely servants; we have done no more than our duty" (Luke 17:10).

In attempting to be meek, we must, as Patanjali tells us, disregard the chatter and the static of external pressures; we must turn silently to the quiet melody playing within us—and within every human heart. In thus responding to our own true nature, we disengage ourselves from discordant distractions and begin to hear the music of the spheres gently turning within us and all about us, in exquisite beauty. Then, as we become sensitive to it softly directing and guiding us, we let ourselves be carried by its soothing currents, and as we become more fully attuned, all our words become a song of love and every motion a dance of joy. Our expression flows out of what fills our hearts. We have become synchronized with the vibratory patterns of the universe whose energy moves the stars and molecules and thus supports the manifest world. We are instruments for the expression of this delightful music, and we have only to prepare ourselves to allow it to flow through us as clearly and strongly as we possibly can.

When we become pure enough for it to be able to flow through us smoothly, we begin to resonate with each subtle and refined innuendo of the melody. The universal pattern and our own become identical; we are one. Our meekness thereby yields the confidence, energy and skill of an artist at work, and in the process of allowing higher beauty to flow through us, we ourselves become beautiful. This blissful union is the very essence of yoga synthesis and integration, for on the mystic plane there are no polarities, opposites or limiting boundaries.

Just as a perfect instrument can become a channel for expressing truly universal themes, so can we become instruments for creating the work of the higher will by accepting our limitations, refining our skills and performing our duties as well as we can. Being meek requires the faith that the music of the universe is progressing as it should and that we are a small, though integral, part of its unfolding. Jesus said that faith the size of a mustard seed could move mountains. Surely, then, through being meek in the full sense of the word, we will be able to gain control over our own life situations. In becoming faithful instruments for the higher will, we become a part of the resounding orchestra playing the universal melody and flow in harmony with its direction, true to our own nature and purpose. Thus the meek whom Jesus speaks of in this Beatitude permeate the world with gentle strength. Their energy eventually determines the course of events, and so the world is theirs.

VI

Blessed are they which do hunger and thirst after righteousness. . . .

The fourth Beatitude, "Blessed are they which do hunger and thirst after righteousness: for they shall be filled" (Matt. 5:6), offers more than just reassurance to the spiritual aspirant; it provides instruction to all those who seek happiness. It also embodies the essence of Jesus' psychology, representing the best counsel he can give to us as we learn to resolve our personal problems and ease our suffering. In this Beatitude Jesus tells us that satisfaction and fulfillment can be attained by striving for that which is right, or justice. But what is justice, and how do we find it? Justice often seems to be rare, and many times we feel unfairly treated. Why can't we get what we want, and why do others seem to have it so much better than we do even when they seem less deserving?

The Bible offers many teachings on the meaning of justice, clarifying exactly what is intended by the word and explaining how we can benefit by this knowledge in our daily lives. Jesus said, "Do not judge, and you will not be judged yourselves. . . . because the judgments you give out are the judgments you will be given back" (Luke 6:37-38), and, "If you forgive others their failings, your heavenly father will forgive you yours; but if you do not forgive others their failings, your heavenly Father will not forgive your failings either" (Matt. 6:14-15), and, "The amount you measure out is the amount you will be given" (Matt. 7:2).

The biblical idea of justice, then, is different from the law of man, and it is interesting to see that these biblical references closely parallel the concept that, in yoga psychology, is called the law of *karma*. According to this wretches will eventually create wretchedness for themselves, and those who have led good and just lives will eventually be rewarded a hundredfold. However, this is not a literal "eye for an eye" attitude. It is the law of absolute and perfect justice by which we must always face the consequences of our own actions; we get what we deserve. If we must pay a *karmic* debt, retribution may not be apparent on this temporal, physical plane or in this lifetime alone; it may take many incarnations. But the wretches of the past can definitely become the saints of the future, though it may take centuries upon centuries of work and pain and learning in order for the transformation to completely take place.

Given this expansive view of life and inner transition, it is easy to see that impressions gleaned from overt cues may oftentimes be deceiving. Just as one person may appear to be holy, and yet actually be quite unscrupulous, so also may one seem to have been given all the world can offer, and still be miserable. Likewise, one such as the wandering *sadhu* of India, who by worldly standards is a subject for pity, may actually be filled with wisdom and bliss. Even the misfit, or underdog, may find a place of glory, for as the Bible says, "It was the stone rejected by the builders that became the keystone" (Matt. 21:42).

Real justice and reward cannot be objectively viewed from the manifest plane, since that which is real is not limited to a form or a name. We cannot see the whole picture because universal justice is balanced within a more subtle, long-range concept of existence than we are now able to perceive. Jesus said, "Your Father who sees all that is done in secret will reward you" (Matt. 6:4). However, he "causes the sun to rise on bad men as well as good" (Matt. 5:45).

In actuality, according to the law of *karma* each of us attracts exactly what is due to us, and this is exactly what we need for our own development. It is for us, of course, to perceive why or how we have earned what we have from our current actions and how to use this awareness for our betterment. Thus, when we keep our eyes turned toward the unchanging reality of the beyond, we can realize that every daily situation can be an opportunity to develop the desired traits which are now deficient in ourselves. Such self-observation and self-analysis are characteristic practices in yoga psychology. So rather than being aggrieved at injustice, we can always cultivate the good in every turn of events.

There is a story of a traveling monk, for example, who begged for his food. One day his teacher asked him, "What will you do if the people give you slop?"

He replied, "I will thank them for not giving me ashes."

"What if they give you nothing?"

"I will be grateful for the opportunity to fast."

"And if they stone you?"

"I will thank them for not killing me outright."

"And what if they do kill you," his teacher asked.

"Then I should be grateful to them for liberating me from this mortal form so I can be with God," came the final response.

Cheerfulness, then, is a matter of choice, not of circumstance. We are not helpless victims; we are creative builders—for better or worse, and if we keep a cheerful, childlike, awareness of the infinite truth, no temporary, unreal phenomena can affect our happiness.

According to yoga psychology, our personal transformation begins on the thought plane, and when we look for the positive, the positive is what we find. "Clean the inside of the cup and dish first so that the outside may become clean as well" (Matt. 23:26), said Jesus. Thus, our inner and outer personalities become identical, and our thoughts become manifest. According to yoga psychology, outside occurrences are merely an expression of inner thoughts and beliefs, and negative thoughts and emotions lead only to suffering. In this way, a poor self-image becomes a self-fulfilling prophecy, and we remain trapped in our limiting ego boundaries.

On the other hand Jesus said, "Everything you ask for, believe that you have it already, and it will be yours" (Mark 11:24). We have the free will and responsibility to develop whatever we want for ourselves, and if we can control our thoughts and cultivate the desired mental habits, or patterns, then their outer manifestations will follow. By understanding the universal law of cause and effect and the power of thought, we can attain whatever we strive for.

The key point is, what do we really want? What do we hunger and thirst for? If we feed ourselves candy, then we will not want a well balanced meal—our appetite will be spoiled. Similarly, if we want only mundane, or transient, pleasures, then our hunger for the real, permanent joys of existence will be spoiled. Likewise, if we overdo even a good thing, this extremism will make us sick. Those who are appeased with worldly objects or praise alone, for instance, have "had their reward"; they have no real appetite, or they have curbed it with junk food, and so they go unnourished and suffer from lack of spiritual nutrients. Those who seek only spiritual fulfillment, however, are given exactly what they need for continued inner development.

Thus, we each get exactly what we desire. We make our own choice. What could be more fair? The trick is to hold out for the main course. This is especially difficult, living as we do in the supermarket of modern America where there are so many enticing treats and advertisements. We must be discriminating, determined and patient in order to get the food that will really nourish our spirits and satisfy us with eternal vitality.

To be thirsty for the truth is to be receptive and open. Then, like a plant, we can absorb as much as our capacity permits. If our hunger is boundless, then so is the truth, and only by it can we be filled. So to be truly happy we must develop a raging hunger and a burning thirst for the eternal, universal truth. As a drowning person seeks air and thinks only of this one all-pervading desire, so should we strive for the real. Our appetizers are the spiritual disciplines we practice—remembering the light within, meditating, loving others. Jesus tells us to listen to his words, and act on them. By the same token, yoga psychology tells us that positive action must follow positive thought. Our empathy and love for others are expressed to them through our words and behavior.

Thinking positively, cultivating peace of mind and being just to others will bring us in harmony with the vibrations of the universal law. Jesus encouraged us to follow the spirit rather than the letter of the law when he said, "The Sabbath was made for man, not man for the Sabbath" (Mark 2:27), and, "What I want is mercy, not sacrifice" (i.e., ritual) (Matt. 9:13), and, "Alas for . . . you who pay your tithe. . . and have neglected the weightier matters of the Law— justice, mercy, good faith" (Matt. 23:23). He did not abide by human regulations, or traditions, or lip service, but lived in wholehearted love for humanity and the higher will. Neither did he overtly advocate strong political action per se. He said "Give back unto Ceasar what belongs to Ceasar—and to God what belongs to God" (Luke 20:25). His seemed to be a politics of service to humanity and of inner growth. Helping others is a manifestation of this inner politics, and to do this we must first be strong and loving in helping ourselves. So too, yoga psychology is a nonritualistic science, dealing primarily with personal transformation.

Jesus told us that the greatest commandment is to love God above all and to love our neighbors as ourselves. "Always treat others as you would like them to treat you; that is the meaning of the law" (Matt. 7:12), he said. Jesus provided detailed instructions on how to live by this, the Golden Rule, and thereby gain justice and happiness. "Love your enemies," he said, "do good to those who hate you, bless those who curse you, pray for those who treat you badly. To the man who slaps you on one cheek, present the other cheek too. . . . Give to everyone who asks you, and do not ask for your property back from the man who robs you" (Luke 6:27-30), and, "If anyone wants to borrow, do not turn away" (Matt. 5:42), and, "Lend without any hope of return. You will have a great reward . . . for the Most High is himself kind to the ungrateful and wicked" (Luke 6:35). This is strikingly similar to one of the basic tenets of karma yoga which is that we must do our work selflessly, with no thought of reward.

How petty the little worries and dreams of daily life seem when viewed from this broad and loving perspective. From this standpoint, the things of the manifest world appear as mere playthings to be used by us, as children would, for our own learning and enjoyment. How foolish it then feels to compare one person to another when our inner needs and abilities, based on our own past actions, are so unique and diverse. If we were all treated exactly the same way, *that* would be the great injustice, for some would be stifled and others overwhelmed.

The law of *karma*, as expressed in Jesus' words, maintains the universal justice which satisfies our every desire and which alone can fulfill us. This justice is all-pervading, eternal and true. So if we see justice from this broad perspective and live by the law of *karma* and the Golden Rule, if we are truly righteous in the biblical sense of the word, we will gain true happiness and peace of mind.

VII

Blessed are the merciful. . . .

The fifth Beatitude, "Blessed are the merciful: for they shall obtain mercy" (Matt. 5:7), is the foundation of Jesus' philosophy. It is one of his major contributions to the evolution of the human race, for the moral outlook expressed in this short statement replaces the old law of reciprocity (an eye for an eye) with the more highly developed law of love (turn the other cheek). This high moral code is the basis of Jesus' major psychological guidelines for improving human relations; through it he implies that we may enhance our interaction with others and obtain a healthy state of mind by consciously implementing the cause/effect quality of mercy in our daily lives.

Defining mercy as charity, love or what in yoga psychology is called *ahimsa* (active non-injury) helps us to appreciate the full value of its possible impact on our personalities, for it entails much more than merely feeding the hungry

or nursing the sick. It must be an essential principle in every aspect and moment of our lives if
we are to attain true peace of mind and happiness.

Love alone has the power to transform ourselves and our world; negative emotions and
selfish actions only generate further negativity
and isolation. But love does not come to us of
itself; it must be created within and earned from
others as a reaction to our own loving behavior
and thoughts.

Living in relationship with others constitutes
the very fabric of life, but making this into a
productive interaction is a challenging art, requir-
ing constant sensitivity to the needs and reactions
of others as well as astute observation of our own
thoughts and actions. Expecting companionship
from others, without initiating loving action,
only leads to frustration and loneliness. Conversely, by being a friend to others, by seeking
out ways to make them happy, we will find
friends and happiness coming to us. The way to
make a friend is to be a friend; the way to gain
love is to give love. This is also an expression of
the ancient law of *karma*; what we receive is what
we offer.

So Jesus tells us that by moving outside ourselves and being concerned with the well-being of
others, we, in turn, will be provided for. In other
words, when we feel like unloved, persecuted
victims and dwell in self-doubt and condemnation, the way out is not to analyze the situation

endlessly, nor is it to make others change; it is, rather, to look for ways to have greater empathy and love for those around us. Therefore, shifting the focus from ourselves to others paradoxically places the locus of control within ourselves. Rather than being victims, we are then in control, making positive choices and taking positive action.

Selfish people are not merciful; they will not hesitate to hurt others in order to meet their own selfish ends. Mercy is based on selflessness, and it expands the personality; the lack of mercy contracts the personality. Love begets love, but even a "righteous" hatred of evil will raise a wave of hatred and evil in our own minds.

Jesus said, "Offer the wicked man no resistance" (Matt. 5:39), and he also tells us that peace is attained by cultivating indifference toward the wicked and compassion for the unhappy. Likewise, Patanjali, in the Yoga Sutras, states that undisturbed calmness of mind is attained by practicing friendliness for the happy, compassion for the unhappy, delight in the virtuous and indifference toward the wicked.

If we have been unjustly accused by the wicked or ignorant our innocence will eventually become evident by our own behavior, but to condemn our accusers gives them evidence of our own lack of mercy. Jesus said, "Forgive them; they do not know what they are doing" (Luke 23:24), and it is only when we fully empathize with and forgive others that we can ourselves obtain forgiveness. If we condemn others, we surely condemn ourselves as well and will, in turn, draw the criticism of others. Jesus' teachings on this topic in the Sermon on the Mount are an excellent illustration of the yoga law of *karma*.

Mercy is based on selflessness. By drawing our attention away from ourselves and from negativity through the practice of mercy, our personal boundaries expand to include all others, and we are thereby embraced and enveloped in the yoga universal Self, or the Christian mystical body. Jesus said, "Even as you do to the least of these, so you do unto me" (Matt. 25:40), and, "So always treat others as you would like them to treat you" (Matt. 7:12). According to this point of view, then, we are all cells in the body of humanity; there is only one of us. Understanding this, Jesus acted as a never-ending flow of mercy, dedicating himself, with infinite patience and forgiveness, to serving those who suffer here. Considering the plight of others and inventing ways to provide a gentle breeze of love in their lives brightens our own lives as well. On the other hand, to withhold mercy from another is to withhold it from ourselves and to block contact with the Self, or God. Thus, the errors and suffering of others give us the opportunity to take creative initiative in performing the altruistic practices of love and service, and this in turn is therapeutic to our own development.

Frequently, however, it seems as if we direct negative energy to an already injured area when we dwell on a single fault no matter how many proper actions we have performed previously or how many other redeeming qualities still exist. Or sometimes a feeling of inferiority causes us to project a false sense of our own superiority, and we criticize others in an attempt to make ourselves seem better by comparison. Interestingly enough, however, the shortcomings of others which are the most irksome to us are generally those which are probably the most apparent in ourselves—although we may not be aware of it.

A negative reaction to another's behavior, then, can act as an indicator of areas we ourselves need to work on. For example, if we find ourselves quick to criticize another's tendency to be greedy, perhaps we are angry that the other person is actually manifesting our own suppressed, or latent, desire, even though we may not be conscious of this. Whereas we could be grateful to others for acting as mirrors and helping us to recognize our own hang-ups, our egos simply cannot cope with that hated facet of our own selves. And so we assume the worst and impute bad motives to another because our own conscience is not clear. Sometimes it is just too hard to admit that the irritating actions of others are also tendencies dwelling within ourselves.

Recognizing this, Jesus pointed out that we

all have shortcomings, and we would do better to "take the plank out of our own eye first," so we can see clearly before we criticize a splinter in our neighbor's, (Matt. 7:5). He also said, "If there is one of you who has not sinned, let him be the first to throw a stone" (John 8:7). These enemies, be they other people or our own intra-psychic blocks, point out the areas in which we need help, and we can appreciate them for serving this function.

Our faults are not barriers, but indicators which present us with the opportunity to improve our direction. Perhaps if we could learn to empathize with and forgive our unsuccessful attempts to imitate perfection, we could also learn to forgive these unproductive negative tendencies in ourselves and others.

The habit of seeing the negative in others makes us dwell on our own negativity, and we then spiral downward into self-condemnation, hatred, envy and depression. Negative thoughts act as a poison. It is much more effective to affirm the positive aspects in ourselves and others and to optimistically and steadily continue onwards. As we love ourselves, so will we love others, accepting all and excluding none.

Mercy toward ourselves, then—total unconditional self-acceptance and self-forgiveness—is essential for nurturing spiritual growth and for relating well to others. Yoga psychology, too, emphasizes the emotional mental tone we should foster rather than the faults we may commit. The important point is to maintain a peaceful, balanced, open and loving state of mind. If we decide that the effects of an action are disruptive to this, then we should experiment with alternative responses to discover reactions which will allow us to remain truly calm and merciful.

Another technique which may help us remain merciful is to take care only of this moment. That is enough to deal with. If we ride the crest of the instant openly, with full love and awareness, making it the best we possibly can, then the future will take care of itself—for it is present actions which comprise the future and on which future reactions depend. As Jesus said, "Neither do I condemn you. Go away and don't sin any more" (John 7:11). The thing to do after a fall is to simply get up and continue on, resolving to be more aware, conscientious and determined.

Paul tells us that the greatest of all the attributes is charity—which is often translated as mercy, and as love. Love for others, love for ourselves and love for God is one and the same thing, for it is not the target of our actions, but the process of acting, which generates this quality in us. We do not have to find a leper colony or a den of iniquity in order to serve the downtrodden. We have only to learn to have mercy on ourselves so that we can give that love to others—and we can love others only to the extent that we love ourselves.

VIII

Blessed are the pure in heart. . . .

The sixth Beatitude, "Blessed are the pure in heart: for they shall see God" (Matt. 5:8), expresses the entirety of Jesus' teachings in the most succinct form. This one simple and profound message can work like a *mantra* in our hearts, like a seed in fertile soil, like a culture in milk. It can transform us if we let go, sit quietly and allow it to work. By surrendering ourselves to its power, we can be drawn naturally toward it like iron shavings toward a magnet, for it is the expression of our true nature. Practicing it can ultimately dissipate all the internal pollution which clouds our vision of the perfection within us.

Negativity and condemnation are the inner contaminants that block the smooth flow of peace and joy which should be constantly ours. But in our unhappiness, it often seems that if we are not condemning ourselves, we are condemning others, and we seesaw back and forth from these two extremes, either directing criticism at others through hatred and anger, or at ourselves through guilt and depression. Seldom do we stop long enough to become aware of the stillness of love within which is the strong fulcrum of our existence.

Numerous metaphors have been offered by spiritual teachers throughout the ages to help people realize this center of purity and love within. Jesus told his disciples to come to him as little children, fully receptive in trust, love and spontaneity. Patanjali says that when the mind is purified and concentrated it is completely clear like a lake, or a crystal, from which all heterogeneous particles have been removed. When the modifications of the mind are controlled, he says, then the seeker is established in his own essential nature.

There are a variety of methods for ridding ourselves of the impurities which impair our spiritual progress. These go far beyond cleansing ourselves of the contaminants of the body created by diet or abuse. As Jesus said, "What goes into the mouth does not make a man unclean; it is what comes out of the mouth that makes him unclean" (Matt. 15:11) and, "For from the heart come evil intentions" (Matt. 15:19). So it is on the more subtle plane of thought and feeling that we must ultimately work to purify ourselves.

Paul said, "What makes a man righteous is not obedience to the Law, but faith" (Gal. 2:16). Thus, although very important, good actions are only the outward sign of the inner foundation of personal development; they can be deceiving, or even empty, without a solid base on the more subtle level of our true intentions and desires. We must therefore confront the negative impressions within and then let them flow out to leave ourselves cleansed and refreshed. "Let your behavior change, modeled by your new mind" (Rom. 12:2), Paul tells us. Just as we bathe every morning, so should we take time regularly to wash the heart and mind clean of all disturbing impressions.

The major yogic intervention for accomplishing this is regular meditation. If we don't like what is inside, why should we store it there? We can let it flow out by objectively observing it and by appropriately expressing it. In stillness we can become aware of our internal "pollution" and of the clear perfection hidden beneath it. This is our true identity, for we are all made in the image and likeness of that perfection; when we realize that, all else fades away. The Yoga Sutras say that yoga is the control of the thought-waves in the mind, and the Bible directs, "Be still and know that I am God" (Psalm 46:10). By concentrating on the one clear image of our inner divinity, we gravitate toward it, and we eventually become the manifestation of it. This metamorphosis takes place by clinging to the pure, by concentrating only on that single truth. In such concentration we are not disturbed by the distracting thoughts which may plague us like a swarm of flies. Instead, focusing our attention on the positive rather than on the negative, and applying this attitude to selfless and skillful action allows our inner purity to shine through, and we actually become that image of perfection.

But this transformation is not always a painless process. Crystals are made clear by prolonged pressure, metal is made strong by being well tempered, butter is clarified by being boiled and skimmed, a stone is made into a beautiful form by the harsh blows of the chisel and mallet, and people are made into saints by discipline, self-confrontation, and non-attachment. Jesus tells us, "Every branch that does bear fruit, he prunes to make it bear even more" (John 15:2), and, "Unless a wheat grain falls on the ground and dies, it remains only a single grain; but if it dies, it yields a rich harvest" (John 12:24). This practice of extinguishing the disruptive pull of the ego and senses is also a major facet of yoga psychology.

There is a certain joy in this giving up of attachments, this honesty and this acceptance of duty, however, which makes life light and sweet. An attitude of, "Let your will be done, not mine" (Luke: 22:42) can relieve us of a great burden and release vast energy, bringing a childlike simplicity and enthusiasm to our lives. If a train is on the track, for instance, progress is sure and steady, for there is no resistance; all its efforts are directed to only one task. But if the train is derailed it sinks into a rut, or hits a rock, or overturns. It can proceed no farther. Its true nature is to cling steadfastly to the rails, and when it goes counter to this purpose it meets with conflict and failure.

Sometimes, though, even when we are moving along the track, our progress may seem almost imperceptible, and we tire, wondering when we will surmount the heights. On a steep incline we sometimes have to pause to get up steam or take a spiral route or go just as fast as we can merely to stay in the same place. But these up-hill hauls are essential if we are to reach the clear vista at the top. Perseverance and optimism can see us through these struggles as can one-pointed dedication to the final goal and implicit trust in the path. As Jesus said, "Your endurance will win you your lives" (Luke 21:19), and this is closely related to the concentration and devotion described in yoga psychology. Our inner voice, called *buddhi*, or conscience, will tell us the way if we will only listen to it and trust it.

The power of positive thinking is so dynamic that identifying ourselves with the strength and purity within can make this actually become a self-fulfilling prophesy. Jesus said that faith the size of a mustard seed can move mountains (Matt. 17:20). Conversely, since the thoughts and the emotions are inextricably linked, if our attention constantly dwells on self-recrimination or judgmental criticism, then we will likewise feel worthless. But if we continuously cultivate gentle and forgiving thoughts, then feelings of love and hope will blossom. The Proverbs say, "As a man thinketh in his heart, so is he" (Prov. 23:7).

In the long run it is actually easier to accept the task at hand, to confront the conflict within and to be loving in relationships with others than it is to go off the track into negativity or to deny our true potential for success. This detour can only lead us to treacherous terrain where we may wallow in frustration, unhappiness and despair. If it is difficult to travel on rough surfaces, then it makes sense for us to avoid the areas where the bogs and pitfalls lie and to adhere to the "straight and narrow" path which leads to the view we seek.

In this life there is a steady line of "visitors" seeking admission to our hearts and minds, each knocking more frantically than the next. These are the desires and distractions which disturb us from working toward our goal of purification. They will persist if we open the door to them, even if it is to tell them to go away, but if we simply allow these distractions to knock and refrain from responding to them, they will eventually tire, give up and go away. This is one meaning of what the yogis called non-attachment—the state in which one does not get hooked by tempting or aggravating intrusions. We simply let them pass. Then we will hear only the quiet, rhythmic tapping of our own pure hearts. If we entertain only that one guest within, the others will realize that there is simply no place for them.

Such a process of observance and non-attachment is the very essence of yoga meditation, the major technique for attaining inner purity. In meditation we allow the various thoughts, desires, sensations, memories, plans to rise to our awareness and we witness them. Sitting in steady calmness, we watch these diverse intrusions as if we were observing a stream flowing by, or a line of traffic or a parade of horses. We don't jump in and float away, or hitch a ride, or lasso anything. We neither grasp nor reject, no matter what comes by. We simply observe, and if we lose our concentration, we gently return to our point of focus, usually a sound or a *mantra*.

Yoga psychology teaches that this practice will allow the heterogeneous, distracting thoughts to dissipate as we reinforce, by constant awareness, the homogeneous focus of our concentration. Thus the internal pollution clouding our true nature is replaced by a clear, clean and pure substance, and we eventually realize our true inner nature, the Self. When the heart is purified in this way there is no filmy obstruction blocking our vision of the divine reality dwelling therein, and we see God.

IX

Blessed are the peacemakers. . . .

The seventh Beatitude, "Blessed are the peacemakers, for they shall be called children of God" (Matt. 5:9), could be interpreted as Jesus' praise for those who settle arguments. But looking deeper, it becomes apparent that the real peacemakers are probably those who have made peace with themselves. The mere presence of such individuals radiates an aura of peace which has a calming, uplifting effect on those around them. They have made peace within, and their spiritual joy flows out to inspire all who do not willfully block it. So powerful is the influence of the presence of a peaceful child of God, such as Jesus, that many people sought only to touch the hem of his robe, and others were pleased merely to sit silently at his feet.

When his disciples asked him who was the greatest in the kingdom of heaven, Jesus called a little child over to him and said to them, "I tell you solemnly, unless you change and become like little children, you will never enter the kingdom of heaven. And so, the one who makes himself as this little child is the greatest in the kingdom of heaven" (Matt. 18:3-4). On another occasion he said, "I bless you, Father, Lord of heaven and of earth, for hiding these things from the learned and the clever and revealing them to mere children" (Matt. 11:25).

What is it about the nature of little children that would warrent such striking remarks? What characteristics can we infer from this Beatitude that we should emulate if we are to become children of God?

We have all experienced the joy of watching children at play, and few can resist the charm of the carefree toddler. Children have perennially provided a ray of light in even the bleakest conditions, and thus they are truly a gift to humanity with all its troubles. Little children usually seek to do that which pleases their parents, and they strive to be like them in every way. They have no worries over the things of the world, for they know their parents will provide for all their needs. They do not fret about the future nor do they cling to the past, for they rest assured that they will be bathed in guiding, forgiving, parental love—and that is what matters most to them.

Little children do not constantly connive to plan a certain end, but with spontaneity and abandon they follow their nature and intuition to respond appropriately to each new moment. They sing and dance; they cry out and laugh just as the spirit moves them. They are unabashed about expressing their needs openly, and they accept their emotions. In their innocence and purity, they remain ever open to others, ever trusting and receptive. Their vulnerability is also their strength, however, for it invites a loving response and permits them to learn from their environment by making mistakes. Toddlers somehow take it in stride that there will be many falls before they master walking. They respond to their internal promptings naturally; when they are sleepy, they sleep; when they are hungry, they eat. They do not feel shame or criticize unjustly. They are openly loving and openly enraged.

Submitting themselves to the discipline of their parents when their will does not coincide with that of their superiors, little children eventually adapt their behavior to the parent, but in doing so they do not give up their own integrity, their right to question and disagree or their attempts to find another means for getting their own way if possible. They experiment with themselves and their environment, discovering what gives joy and what gives pain.

Little children have complete faith that their needs will be met. Having simple tastes, they revel in appreciation of the ordinary—a shiny pebble, a kind glance. They perform every action with full concentration on that act; nothing exists except their interaction with the present moment.

Their smiles and their touches come easily, and they act with unself-conscious confidence. They are simultaneously poised and clumsy; even their *faux pas* are endearing.

Having no concept of dishonesty, their motives are beyond reproach and their expressions beyond question. Little children are so pure that they cannot hide anything or respond in an artificial way; social norms mean nothing to them. They teach others a great deal by reflecting their behavior and by responding directly to their actions. They learn rapidly, find comfort easily and are absolutely true to their inner nature. No wonder Jesus said, "Let the little children come to me. . . for it is to such that the kingdom of God belongs" (Matt. 10:14).

Reviewing these attributes of little children, it is understandable that they are cherished so and that Jesus held them as exemplary models for the spiritual seeker. But the children of God of which Jesus speaks are an even more priceless boon to humankind, for these are the bright beings who maintain the most admirable qualities of little children while attaining full spiritual maturity. Thus, they provide a precious source of joy for all who come in contact with them. These beings have surrendered themselves to the higher powers, and with the loving trust of a child for its mother, they have placed themselves in the lap of God.

There is a difference, however, between being

childish and being childlike. All of the great
spiritual teachers have been childlike in many
ways. Living their lives simply and honestly,
with complete faith and love, they act openly
and spontaneously, viewing the objects of the
world as their toys, the chain of events as a
game; having overcome all conflicts and distractions, and having made peace with themselves,
they find their peace within. In the presence of
one such as this we can realize our own childlike nature and can more easily let go of the
restricting burdens assumed by the ego in its
childish attempts to be grown up. How much
easier it is to play our lives as children of God and
live in peace than it is to be the rebellious ado-
lescent or the inflexible, strict adult.

Having attained a highly evolved state of
conscious "childhood," Jesus was able to leave
his disciples with these words: "Peace I bequeath
to you, my own peace I give you. . . . Do not let
your hearts be troubled or afraid" (John 14:27).
Thus do the children of God create peace in the
world.

X

*Blessed are they which are persecuted
for righteousness' sake. . . .*

he eighth Beatitude, "Blessed are they
which are persecuted for righteousness sake: for
theirs is the kingdom of heaven" (Matt. 5:10),
tends to conjur up images of martyrs in torment,
and this was indeed the plight of many of the
early followers of Jesus. But we may wonder
what message this saying holds for us today when
there is no such pogrom being executed. Surely it
is still relevant, for in a world as materialistically
and rationally oriented as the one in which we
live, spiritual considerations are not uncommonly
disregarded or smothered, and those who reach
for the farther limits of human experiencing are
frequently either ridiculed as being goofy or
dismissed as being fanatics—and sometimes this
may indeed be the case.

But there are, as well, many sincere and level-
headed seekers who are victims of this prejudice.
Paul cautions, "Do not model yourselves on the

behavior of the world around you" (Rom. 12:2), but the non-spiritual have difficulty understanding the goals and practices of those who are striving to go beyond the material, rational world, and they are sometimes condescending, or even hostile, toward them. Then, too, many have trouble discriminating between those who are eccentric for perversity's sake and those who are unconventional for righteousness' sake. In this Beatitude Jesus specifies that those who seek what is right and just, be it howsoever unpopular, are the blessed ones. Merely being persucuted does not bring grace; many bring torment upon themselves by their own obstinance.

Throughout the ages there has been a recurring pattern of mixed admiration and antagonism for mystics. Perhaps the masses are jealous of the greater strength and contentment that very highly evolved people display, or maybe they view nonconformity as slightly pathological, or perhaps they become more acutely aware of their own shortcomings in the presence of more fully integrated personalities. The realization that they may be missing out on fulfilling their own capacity can be very painful, and so, to compensate, they may become defensive or try to lash out in anger, fear or denial toward those whose lives threaten them.

Because of the different course they have chosen, and because of the tendency others have to segregate them, high achievers, be it in intellectual, creative or spiritual concerns, are frequently lone wolves, living rather isolated lives and sharing their innermost selves only with the few who can understand them. This reclusive existence, however, can actually serve to enhance the ability of spiritual seekers to attain their goals. This is not to say that such people do not participate with others in the stream of life. On the contrary, they are frequently compelled to experience intensely the paradoxes of life. But they always seem to embrace some measure of asceticism, at least at the onset of their quest, for their purpose requires discipline and sacrifice.

This has always been true of those following the spiritual path. The values, practices and sensory withdrawal described by Patanjali, for instance, are prerequisites for meditation and spiritual growth in raja yoga. Such seekers lead simple lives, free from most everyday distractions, so they can focus their energy more effectively. They realize that their actions may set them apart, possibly causing them to be resented, but they choose to follow their higher promptings rather than the sometimes spiritually restrictive norms of society. Jesus was not concerned with human approval; he did not "break away from the commandment of God for the sake of . . . tradition" (Matt. 15:3).

Jesus told the apostles, "Because you do not belong to the world . . . the world hates you" (John 15:19), and because they are disliked, some nonconformists may react with disdain to conventional members of society. They consider themselves to be members of an elite. But self-righteousness has nothing to do with being righteous. Others are petty and superficial only when we define them as such and only if we behave in that way, ourselves, for we all hold the jewel of divinity in our hearts.

This is clearly set forth in yoga psychology as it is in Jesus' advice to "pray for those who persecute you" (Matt. 5:44). To do so keeps us in touch with this reality and with our higher motivational force. Any emotional response creates a visceral reaction and lowers us to the level of animal instincts, thus cutting off any possibility of our experiencing an expanded state of consciousness. In the midst of his own persecution Jesus said, "Forgive them; they do not know what they are doing" (Luke 23:34). The immediate reward of such a stance is continued contact with total peace, or the "kingdom of heaven." The righteous response to persecution is love.

People who are persecuted in the process of moving toward their own inner destiny accept the rebukes of others, for this strengthens their resolution and willpower. Thus Jesus said, "Alas for you when the world speaks well of you" (Luke 6:26). To take a stance with conviction requires the ability to put up with criticism, for someone will always disagree, but one who endures hardship rather than abandon his or her beliefs is happier than one who yields such beliefs rather than suffer. Jesus also said, "Anyone who loves his life shall lose it; anyone who hates his life in this world will keep it for the eternal life" (John 12:25). There is pleasure in courageously accepting such a challenge, particularly when we know it will benefit others whom we love.

Many spiritual traditions emphasize the need for seekers to go through a purgative stage in which their desires are burned away through altruistic discipline, for it is said that one who endures the strokes of the chisel is shaped into the form of the deity. For this reason mystics have traditionally utilized sublimation, making use of the austerities and tasks meted out to them and chosing not to gratify the lower desires of their senses or ego. Ritualistically, an offering is purified in the sacrificial fires, and so without some amount of sacrifice there is no purification. Likewise, without perseverence there is no benefit.

Jesus said, "Happy are those who are persecuted in the cause of right" (Matt. 5:10). Miserable are those who hedonistically seek joy from temporal, transitory and superficial pleasures, because they are always left unsatiated and disappointed. These pleasures are fleeting and do not appease our innermost craving for deep, permanent happiness. No wonder, then, when we cannot find true satisfaction even in pleasure, that some are bewildered and resentful toward those who can somehow find peace in the midst of persecution.

But true seekers are neither victims nor masochists. Rather, they look beyond the mundane and the temporal and consciously choose to accept or reject experiences, and they base their decision on one criterion: Will this help me to grow, to be more pure, to be stronger, to be more in touch with my real self? They see every moment as a choice, and being aware of the consequences of their actions, they select for growth. The more they channel their lower promptings, the happier and freer they become. They are neither passive or reactive, but assertive and initiatory. They are not slaves to their desires but have control of their minds and have mastered their senses.

The most trying form of persecution can be that which we inflict upon ourselves. In our efforts to attain right thought and right action, we are constantly harrassed by the incessant promptings of our senses and ego. The lower self constantly badgers us to indulge in every manner of distraction. It fears its own annihilation and resists our efforts to surpass its limits. Clever and persistent, it cajoles and argues, trying to undermine our determination to accept the discipline necessary to attain our purpose. And we allow it to create a flurry of distracting goals and emotions to avoid confronting the deeper issues of ultimate concern.

But there is beauty even in this constant inner turmoil, for only when the symptoms arise can we treat the illness. The sooner these confrontations with our hidden psyche are made, the sooner their power over us can be dissipated and the sooner we can get on to more basic business. The enemies which at first appear so formidable are, in actuality, not so fierce, and when their self-indulgent, disintegrating tendencies are ignored, they eventually tire and relent. According to yoga psychology, tenacious perseverence, optimism and self-confidence are essential in order to overcome these psychic blocks, while sloth, fear and self-recrimination are the greatest hindrances.

If, for example, we feel scattered and have trouble concentrating, it is better to admit this, and instead of forcing ourselves into a strict and rigorous schedule, we should engage in some pleasant hobby. This will gently train us in the skills of concentration. It is easy to pay attention to that which we love, have skill at and find meaningful. Then, when accepted and given healthful and beneficial outlets, our bothersome tendencies can become our allies, aiding us in our journey beyond the limitations and sufferings of this worldly existence.

Great yoga masters use this concept and turn the weaknesses of their pupils into strengths. Then a transformation takes place; rather than being dualistic, like a wild horse with a stern rider, they become integrated. So we can enjoy what was once a troublesome burden and use it to help us on our journey. In this way, what may originally be seen as persecution, unfair hardship or insurmountable temptation can actually be used as a tool for growth. Thus persecution can be a purifying experience, crystallizing our will, stamina, perseverance and control.

XI

Beware of false prophets. . . .

After delivering the Beatitudes, Jesus continued the Sermon on the Mount with, among other things, a discussion of the relationship between the teacher and the disciple. He said, "It is not those who say to me, 'Lord, Lord,' who will enter the kingdom of heaven, but the person who does the will of my Father in heaven" (Matt. 7:21). Here it would seem that Jesus is admonishing those who will not take action themselves, who feign a helpless, dependent stance to him, expecting salvation by his efforts alone. The Beatitudes reinforce this emphasis on strength and self-reliance.

Although at first glance they may seem to encourage more passivity, this is not at all the case, for the behavior Jesus advocates in the Beatitudes requires great faith, strength of character and determination. Jesus is telling his followers to surrender their egos and sensory gratifications, to give up their possessions, to yearn for spirituality, to offer love and peace to all, to purify themselves and to allow themselves to be persecuted. He is asking them to live a life of complete trust and dedication, and it requires tremendous will, effort and fortitude to accomplish this. Throughout the gospels repeated parables address the absolute necessity for resourcefulness and self-reliance. Consider, for example, the man who buried his talents, the women who forgot the oil for their lamps or the servant who was found sleeping. All of these people wanted to be saved despite their lack of assertiveness, energy and preparation. "The spirit is willing, but the flesh is weak" (Matt. 26: 41). Yet no external force punished them for their shortcomings—they punished themselves by not sowing their own good seeds properly. This is the cause/effect relationship of the law of *karma*.

No external force can either save or condemn us. All comes from within. This is reminiscent of the saying, "God helps those who help themselves." Good actions reap good results. The key is in becoming attuned to the intentions of the higher will and acting from these promptings. But how do we know which voice represents this higher direction, which comes from others' injunctions and which speaks from our own limited ego?

Again, the oft-quoted, "Know thyself" and, "Be still and know that I am God" (Psalm 46:10) come to mind. Jesus said to his disciples both, "You are the light of the world" (Matt. 5:14) and, "I am the light of the world" (John 8:12). This might lead us to conclude that the voice of the spiritual master can be found within. This inner *guru* is identified in yoga psychology as the *buddhi*, the guiding wisdom within each of us which reflects the true Self. It is not to be confused with the narrow self-concepts of our personality, or ego identity *(ahamkara)*, nor does it generate from the storehouse of impressions programmed into us by past experiences *(chitta)* and neither is it a direction from our sensory motor impulses *(manas)*. It is the conscience, our highest and most reliable guide to the beyond within, and the more we attune ourselves to its directions and follow them, the more surely will it speak. Listening to it strengthens it, but ignoring it kills it. This voice always has our own best interests at heart, and it is understanding and compassionate in leading us gently yet steadily toward our goal of self-actualization.

But again, how do we differentiate this one voice from the many debating within us as well as from those outside voices which would tell us what to do? Jesus says, "Beware of false prophets. . . . you will be able to tell them by their fruits" (Matt. 7:15-16). These fruits are the quality of the teacher's words, actions and students. Intrapsychically, they are our own thoughts, feelings and behavior. Determining which are false and which are true inner voices may require many experiments, many failures, however, before we can identify the one which, when we act on its words, guides us most surely to our highest potential. These failures are good things, for they indicate to us which direction *not* to go in, and we are then a bit more sure of the path it would be best to take. It takes determined curiosity and a willingness to accept failure to find the way in this matter.

The issue of knowing how to determine the truth for oneself seems to be a particularly trying one for many in this decade of heightened spiritual interest, clouded as it is by so much New Age mumbo-jumbo and cultish brainwashing. Scores of would-be gurus co-exist with the small handful of authentic masters like thorns on a rose bush. So how can we avoid being snared by some quasi-plausible hype which hooks into our own ego deficiencies and hangups? How do we determine if we're merely buying into a system of idealism and escape or accepting a true spiritual path?

The parallels between psychosis and mysticism, between brainwashing and faith, between cultism and religion have been drawn throughout the centuries, and the debate continues. Some contention can even be made that we are all, to some degree, victims of cultural brainwashing imparted by parent, television, church, teacher, peer, employer, spouse, etc. These influences certainly do exact specific ideologies and behavior, and sometimes at very high stakes, yet the more insidious and threatening procedures of real cult indoctrination strike one much more sharply.

Sadly, the dissociated, indecisive, suggestible and submissive cultists seeking their "escape from freedom" are hardly candidates for great spiritual advancement. Yet it is frequently spiritual longing which spurs them to seek answers in the cult. They will not find what they are seeking, however, for conspicuous by their absence in cultists and their leaders are selflessness, self-fulfillment and inner strength. Theirs is a symbiotic relationship; they are dependent on each other, each sucking on the other's neurotic tendencies for survival. This is a case of the "blind leading the blind," and both fall into a pit.

Cultists and their leaders derive their identity, purpose and power externally, from each other, rather than from their own internal spiritual orientation. Their interaction is characterized by desperate clinging to and using of each other, not by love and service. Their growth is stopped. They are not free. Their locus of control is outside themselves, and they do not see that they have choices in thought or action. Gone are the self-confrontation, inner conflict and existential dissatisfaction which spur us to change. Also anesthetized is the spiritual longing which generates us to strive for our deepest potential, for to cultists the questions have apparently been answered and the exact path defined.

Inner seeking seems no longer necessary in this constricted state because the outer environment they have arranged has relieved them of this struggle and its reward. Such a stance is diametrically opposed to the precepts of Patanjali's yoga science which stresses self-reliance, self-exploration, inner seeking and astute self-analysis and discrimination. Yoga, in fact, is often referred to as a self-training program.

Cultists seek power from without, and thus they deny their own intrinsic worth and their inner capacity to manage their own lives. This is the infantile stance of dependency, not the mature stance of self-reliance. Nonetheless, deciding whether we are motivated to seek a teacher because of altruism and spirituality or because of fear and dependency can be a difficult issue resolved only by honest self-study. In the final analysis, no matter how much we would like to opt out of this responsibility or disclaim this fact, we alone can decide how best to live our lives, and only we have the means and competency to carry through the plan. This is one of the major tenets of yoga psychology.

Jesus, too, was careful not to encourage blind adherence to dogma, nor did he savor performing miracles merely to impress would-be followers. He said, "It is an evil and unfaithful generation that asks for a sign!" (Matt. 12:39). Yet there are other methods for determining reliable sources of guidance, and Jesus provides two means for

evaluating human character, be it our own or that
of another. First, he indicated that the eyes show
the light of the soul, and if the eyes shine with
this calm bright light, then there is light within
the person (Matt. 6:22-23). Second, he says, "A
man's words flow out of what fills his heart"
(Matt. 12:34).

Besides observing the light in a teacher and
listening to the quality of his words, other ways
to determine the integrity of a teacher can be
inferred. Taking into consideration the fact that
the Psalm says, "Be still and know that I am God"
(Psalm 46:10), for instance, it follows that those
who "know God" will also have a capacity for
being quite still. In addition, Jesus cautions us
not to be influenced by outside opinions, asking
us how we can believe since we look to one
another for approval, and saying, "Do not keep
judging according to appearances; let your judgment be according to what is right" (John 7:24),
and, "The truth shall make you free" (John
8:32). But how do we know what is right and
true?

The adage, "Know thyself" is the main route
to fulfillment, but this inner knowledge cannot be
discovered by external means such as observing
ourselves in various situations. It comes to us
from ourselves in quiet and stillness. The wisdom
in our own hearts will clearly direct our growth
if we listen to its message. This is the voice of the
buddhi in yoga psychology.

Jesus also says, "No man can be the slave of two masters" (Matt. 6:24), and a true teacher will be free of inner and outer conflict. Integrated people are strong from within, for they are free from dualistic struggles. They know "where they came from and where they are going" (John 8:14), and they can thus be decisive and confident. Their values and purpose are their main motivators, so they are not easily suggestible or dependent. Jesus said, "I am in the Father and the Father is in me" (John 14:10), and "The Father and I are one" (John 10:30), for in him the higher will and the individual person were one and the same. "If you know me, you know my Father too," (John 14:7), he said. Thus, the push/pull of conflict is resolved in quiet stillness and decisive action, in being at one with oneself.

Thus, rather than seeking a parent figure outside ourselves, we can find that support and comfort within us. This is the strength of presence found in advanced individuals and in ourselves during times of peace. Then, Jesus tells us, "Everything now hidden will be made clear" (Luke 12:2), for all that can be known is to be found within. That is why it is called Self-realization.

Yoga psychology states that each individual has the capacity to discover his own inner perfection through sincere and systematic self-study. Although the teacher is an essential guide for the more advanced levels of this search, the student is instructed not to follow him blindly, but to judge his competence for himself. Absolute selflessness is the main criterion the student looks for. But even after the teacher's validity has been determined and the student has made a commitment to study with him, blind faith is not encouraged. Rather, the teacher is viewed as one who has the map to the territory to be traversed, or as a boat to be used in order to cross to the other shore. He can guide, but the student must, in the final analysis, make his own way and learn to discriminate for himself between the true voice of the higher will and the many suggestions and desires which interfere along the way.

The false prophets of ego, instinct and pride arising from within our own experience are perhaps the most difficult ones to identify. Rationales and excuses are hard to perceive for what they are when they originate from within our own mental sets. Our major defenses against their bad advice are sincere self-study, prayer and observance of the results of our own actions; faith in our capacity for and natural tendency toward spiritual growth will keep us from being crippled by the false prophets of doubt and fear.

XII

*Thy kingdom come . . . on earth
as it is in heaven.*

When looked at as a whole, the Sermon on the Mount can be interpreted as a prescription for making a perfect society, one in which the citizens always treat each other as they themselves would like to be treated and in which they surrender to the higher will in love and service. In such a utopian setting love establishes the prime order, and spirituality provides the law and purpose of the people. It is the kingdom of God on earth.

Jesus prophetically proclaimed, "The kingdom of heaven is close at hand" (Matt. 10:7), and his message prepared the followers for a completely new phase of development. Faithfully, they awaited the transformation of the world, the resurrection and second coming, in their own lifetimes, for Jesus had told them, "I have come to complete the Law of the prophets. . . . Not one little stroke shall disappear from the law until its purpose is completed" (Matt. 5:17-18). But such a comprehensive and apocalyptic transition was not to occur as quickly as they had expected, at least not on the collective level. In terms of the total age of humanity, Jesus' message has yet to reach maturity; the seed is still germinating in preparation for its breaking forth.

Although the law of love which Jesus described has not yet been universally established on a societal level, the seed is definitely stirring. As our species evolves we become ever more able to live according to its subtle, spiritual mode. We become more refined and capable of the increasingly delicate strength it requires. Teilhard de Chardin, for instance, describes the current evolutionary phase of humanity as predominantly a development of the spirit—the body and mind having been sufficiently perfected to allow for this.[1] Sri Aurobindo speaks of our age as one of mental subjectivism (which is the presursor of the age of spiritualism),[2] and yoga science reflects similar developmental phases for humanity.

According to the Upanishads, for instance, reality is seen first as material, physical, mechanistic and utilitarian; second, it is appreciated as life, vitalism, expansionism and dynamic mastery;

1   Teilhard de Chardin, *The Phenomenon of Man* (New York: Harper and Row), 1959.
2 Sri Aurobindo, *The Essential Aurobindo* (New York: Schocken Books), 1973.

third, it is mental, intellectual, psychic and intuitive. Last, the realm beyond these is reached, and there is an age of spirituality, of perfect unity in diversity from which the highest powers may be tapped and the purest consciousness attained. Thus, the species moves from object to animal to human to angel. As Jesus said, "At the resurrection, men and women . . . are like the angels in heaven" (Matt. 22:30).

Jesus suggested that we be aware of the "signs of the times," and the current signs of this century, apparent in the works of the great artists and thinkers who constitute the growing tip of humanity's potential, seem to reflect a collective intuition that some transition toward spirituality may in fact be taking place. Science is investigating the thinning walls between matter and energy; the arts are more nonobjective and inner oriented than they have been in the past; philosophy is embracing more idealistic and subjective interpretations of reality; psychology is moving toward the transpersonal and extrasensory aspects of consciousness; religions are less dogmatic and ritualistic and more ecumenical and transcendental than they have been; and politics are becoming more humanistic and globally oriented. Ever-growing numbers of people hold a sense of some impending great occurrence, be it holocaust, visitation from other planets, or regeneration of the species, and the pop culture flaunts this notion with talk of the New Age and the dawning of Aquarian energy. Psychics, artists, mystics, as well as many ordinary citizens, seem to feel that just below the horizon some new aspect of our consciousness is preparing to ascend.

This rising of the spiritual sun is viewed in yoga psychology as the opening of the flow of love; it can occur not only on the collective level but also on an individual level. It is the rising of the vital energy, *kundalini*, through and beyond the centers that are concerned with survival, sensuality and power to the place that is characterized by the giving of unconditional love embodied in the heart. When one resides in this heart level of awareness, one transcends the lower concerns and begins to tap the higher divine energies. This is Teilhard's "divine milieu" on the level of the collective consciousness, and it is the sacred heart of Jesus on the individual level. It represents the best of humanness and godliness and is the platform from which one takes flight spiritually. In instructing his disciples in how to attain this refined level, Jesus told them "not to worry about your life . . . nor about your body" (Matt. 6:25) but to "set your hearts on his kingdom first and on his righteousness, and all these other things will be given as well" (Matt. 6:33). By attaining this subtle level of unconditional selfless love, all else is obtained automatically, and no desires plague one's happiness.

Jesus often referred to a judgment day, or resurrection, when the kingdom of heaven would manifest on earth, when the spirit would become the foundation of reality rather than the material, vital or intellectual forces which now rule the scene. In directing his followers to interpret the signs of the times, he told them, "The kingdom of God does not admit to observation," (Luke 17: 20), and then he said, "You must know, the kingdom of God is among you" (Luke 17:21). To find this spiritual realm, one must look within and perceive with the higher faculties beyond the senses.

Such a transformation must occur within each heart if it is to blossom on a more global scale as well. Jesus is called "the word made flesh," and he can be seen as a high evolutionary, a highly advanced precursor, or a mutant sample, of the potential of the species. He proclaimed that each person has the ability to attain the kingdom of God and that this state dwells within every heart. (Yogis describe this inner divinity as a flame burning in the cave of the heart.) But attaining such an evolution of consciousness on the individual, or genetic, level is not easy. Jesus warns of the deception, conflict, destruction, persecution and sorrow which will precede the change when he says, "The stars will come falling from heaven and the powers in the heavens will be shaken" (Mark, 13:25). But he also says, "You are not to prepare your defense" (Luke 21:14), and "Anyone who tries to preserve his life will lose it" (Luke 17:33). But he then adds, "There is no need to be afraid, little flock, for it has pleased your Father to give you the kingdom" (Luke 12:32).

Yogis refer to this era as *Kali Yuga*, the age of moral decline and destruction, but how is it possible that the destruction and decline of *Kali Yuga* coexists with the blossoming of the new spiritual age which Aurobindo and Teilhard predict? As Dickins might say, it is the best of times; it is the worst of times. Wars, starvation, poverty, disease and insanity threaten us as the outcasts of society live like rats in their holes, desperate and ready to lash out in blind rage. Yet at the same time an increasing number of people are reporting the attainment of deeper and more subtle levels of awareness. Empathy and the expansion of consciousness have become the major concerns of a growing minority, while the world as a whole seems to decay and crumble in hopeless self-destruction.

The poles of nature—death and regeneration— are Siamese twins; like pleasure and pain, they always come paired. It is as if some beautiful *spiritus mundi* may arise from the rotting corpse of our era's troubles, like the phoenix rising from its own ashes to take flight and soar in blazing flames of vibrant life. This seeming holocaust may be our final salvation as a species, for nature will have balance; she will destroy and she will nurture—because growth cannot take place otherwise.

Tumultuous occurrences precede all times of personal and societal transition. Our foundation shifts when important changes take place, and this can be frightening—but it can also herald a time of creative energy and hope. Jesus said, "When these things begin to take place, stand erect and hold your heads high, because your liberation is at hand" (Luke 21:28).

Therefore, rather than worry and fear, we can rejoice in the turmoil which precedes transformation, and we can keep sight of the higher purpose, letting the old and useless scaffolds crumble. As is repeatedly mentioned in Jesus' teachings, it is in "dying" that eternal life is attained. When the "kingdom" comes and the will of the Father is done "on earth as it is in heaven" (Matt. 6:10), then we will acquire our spiritual inheritance and "be perfect even as [our] heavenly Father is perfect" (Matt. 5:48). Then will the purpose and teaching of Jesus be fulfilled, for those who abide in love abide in God, and God in them, and a society which abides in love is called heaven; the kingdom of God on earth.

The Author

Arpita (Joan Harrigan) is a Ph.D. candidate in Counseling Psychology at the Pennsylvania State University. She has worked as a counselor in two university counseling centers and as an instructor of English and art in an alternative secondary school. She holds a M.Ed. in Alternative Education from Indiana University and an M.S. in Counseling from Texas Tech. In addition, she has been a resident at the Himalayan Institute where she studied with Swami Rama and assisted in the completion of several books.

HIMALAYAN INSTITUTE PUBLICATIONS

Living with the Himalayan Masters	Swami Rama
Yoga and Psychotherapy	Swami Rama, R. Ballentine, M.D. Swami Ajaya
Science of Breath	Swami Rama, R. Ballentine, M.D. A. Hymes, M.D.
Emotion to Enlightenment	Swami Rama, Swami Ajaya
Freedom from the Bondage of Karma	Swami Rama
Book of Wisdom	Swami Rama
Lectures on Yoga	Swami Rama
Life Here and Hereafter	Swami Rama
Marriage, Parenthood & Enlightenment	Swami Rama
A Practical Guide to Holistic Health	Swami Rama
Superconscious Meditation	Pandit Usharbudh Arya, Ph.D.
Philosophy of Hatha Yoga	Pandit Usharbudh Arya, Ph.D.
Meditation and the Art of Dying	Pandit Usharbudh Arya, Ph.D.
God	Pandit Usharbudh Arya, Ph.D.
Yoga Psychology	Swami Ajaya
Foundations, Eastern & Western Psychology	Swami Ajaya (ed)
Psychology East and West	Swami Ajaya (ed)
Meditational Therapy	Swami Ajaya (ed)
Diet and Nutrition	Rudolph Ballentine, M.D.
Joints and Glands Exercises	Rudolph Ballentine, M.D. (ed)
Yoga and Christianity	Justin O'Brien, Ph.D.
Science Studies Yoga	James Funderburk, Ph.D.
Homeopathic Remedies	Drs. Anderson, Buegel, Chernin
Hatha Yoga Manual I	Samskrti and Veda
Hatha Yoga Manual II	Samskrti and Judith Franks
Swami Rama of the Himalayas	L. K. Misra, Ph.D. (ed)
Philosophy of Death and Dying	M. V. Kamath
Practical Vedanta of Swami Rama Tirtha	Brandt Dayton (ed)
The Swami and Sam	Brandt Dayton
Sanskrit Without Tears	S. N. Agnihotri, Ph.D.
Psychology of the Beatitudes	Arpita
Theory and Practice of Meditation	Himalayan Institute
Inner Paths	Himalayan Institute
Meditation in Christianity	Himalayan Institute
Faces of Meditation	Himalayan Institute
Art and Science of Meditation	Himalayan Institute
Therapeutic Value of Yoga	Himalayan Institute
Chants from Eternity	Himalayan Institute
Spiritual Diary	Himalayan Institute
Thought for the Day	Himalayan Institute
Himalayan Mountain Cookery	Martha Ballentine
The Yoga Way Cookbook	Himalayan Institute